MW01611386

THIS DAY SO SWEET

A JOURNEY WITH GRACE

SALLY SUE TITTLE

WING AND A PRAYER PRESS
PO BOX 550
SEABECK, WASHINGTON 98380

WWW.AWINGANDAPRAYERPRESS.COM
WWW.THISDAYSOSWEET.COM

Cover design by Tracey Ryan
Artwork by Nancy Ryan

Printed in the United States of America

Library of Congress Control Number 2006932657
ISBN 0-9774050-0-1

First Edition

Wing and A Prayer Press
PO Box 550
Seabeck, Washington 98380

for Sally and Sue
who light the way

Acknowledgments

For her tenacity and heart, without which this book would not exist, thanks to Peggy Astarita.

For her vision and wisdom, from the center of my heart, thanks to Shirley Wiedeman.

For his invaluable assistance, encouragement and faith, to Steve Lantrip, thank you.

And to the one who makes all my days so sweet, thank you to Tracey Ryan.

Contents

Introduction

This is a true story.

In February of 2001 Sally Tittle was diagnosed with throat cancer and in July of that year with recurrent pancreatic cancer. She was 71 years old and had been a teacher for 17 years in the Dallas school district. Her husband had died in 1982 of throat cancer. She had four children, Diane, Sue, Bryant and Becky.

Her daughter, Sue, who had been a nurse for many years, moved in with Sally to be her primary care giver. At the time Sue, herself, was ill with idiopathic pulmonary fibrosis. IPF is a progressive, terminal lung disease of unknown origin, that causes scarring of the lungs. Pulmonary hypertension and respiratory failure are the eventual outcomes. Average survival times are five to six years. Sue required oxygen 24 hours a day.

Along with Sue came a chubby brown dog named Grace Elizabeth who played a key role as night nurse and companion. Two cats, Ringo and Max, were already in residence.

For the next year Sue wrote e-mails to friends and family. This is their journey...

PART ONE
SALLY AND SUE

Sally's children are Diane, Sue, Bryant and Becky.

Diane is married to Gordon and they have a daughter, Jenny.

Bryant's children are Jacob and Sara.

Becky is married to Tom. Debi and Sherri are Becky's children.

Sally's siblings are:

Uncle William (her older brother), married to Aunt MM (stands for Mary Margaret)

Aunt FiFi (her older sister) is married to Uncle Dade. They have a son Stephen.

FEBRUARY 14, 2001

Mom has the needle biopsies scheduled at Baylor for this Friday at 11 a.m. Hopefully by early next week there can be treatment designs made. I will keep you informed. Mom has had several pretty good days and for that I am thankful. Sue

JUNE 19, 2001

I have noticed a change in Mother's voice for months and months. I have pleaded with her to please get it checked out. This is how it started with Daddy. I noticed a change in his voice. He listened to me and went to the doctor as soon as he could. Mother is a little more hard headed. She saw her throat doctor yesterday and he was alarmed with what he saw. I was not there because Mother insisted that she was going alone. He told her that there is a tumor the size of his thumb on her epiglottis. He recommended immediate hospitalization and she would have a temporary trach. Mother told him that he would have to talk to her children. She was so shocked that she didn't want to ask any more questions. At this point she is wanting to weigh all the information and decide whether she wants to go through with any kind of surgical intervention. When I know more, I will let you know. Please keep her in your prayers. Thanks, Sue

JULY 7, 2001

I talked to the doctor's office on Friday about scheduling the surgery. I was more than shocked when the secretary told me it would be on August 10. I told her that date was unacceptable. She's going to speak with the doctor about referring to another doctor if he can't do the surgery any earlier. Mom continues to require a lot of pain medicine and tires easily, but so far, she has been able to maintain a beautiful garden. When I know anymore, I'll let you know. Sue

JULY 9, 2001

Mom's surgery is scheduled for July 18 at noon. This will be outpatient surgery. I am feeling very positive about the outcome. I will let you know when I know more. Sue

JULY 18, 2001

Mom had her surgery today. She is home and her voice is beginning to sound like it's supposed to. She only had the mass removed. We will know what the biopsy is by Monday. The doctor suspects that they will find squamous cell carcinoma. If it is malignant, he will suggest a course of radiation. Removal of the epiglottis would be the second option. Mom's throat will be sore for about a week. She feels blessed and asked that I send her love. Sue

JULY 21, 2001

Courage is fear that has said its prayers—Karl Barth

JULY 24, 2001

The doctor told Mom today that her tumor was squamous cell carcinoma, a particularly invasive type. He feels he got it all, but he advises follow-up treatment. We go to see a specialist on July 30. Treatment options such as radiation or surgery will be discussed. Mother will not lose her voice. We all have a hopeful spirit about this. If I don't respond to any e-mails it is because my computer has the vapors. Sue

AUGUST 1, 2001

I have good news. Dr. L. the specialist we saw Monday, says that with radiation he feels that it is 100% curable. Mom will go to Baylor and have the treatments. I suspect she will start next week. He says that she might develop a slight dry throat, but no other problems. I hope all is well with you and yours. Sue

AUGUST 7, 2001

Mother experienced a rather sudden increase in pain and was having a bloody vaginal discharge this week. I increased her pain meds with marginal results. She saw the doctor today. He didn't have good news. After a brief exam, he told her that he felt like her pelvic mass has eroded into the vaginal wall. He felt that this was a source of the bleeding. He is also concerned about a possible metastasis to the abdomen. She has the CT scan scheduled for tomorrow in hopes of giving us a clearer picture. Mom has an appointment scheduled for Thursday to see Dr. C., a pain specialist, in hopes of getting a better handle on the pain. Her primary doctor feels like all we can do is offer supportive care and pray that Dr. C. can get her pain control to an acceptable level. She is tired from all of this, so she is spending a lot of time in bed. When I find out more Thursday, I will write another note. Thanks for your prayers. Sue

AUGUST 11, 2001

I am sorry for delay in getting this note out. I heard from the doctor Friday evening. He was calling to give me the report from the CAT scan. They verified that the pelvic mass had eroded through the vaginal wall. This was the source of the bleeding. It was also noted that Mom had free-floating fluid in her abdomen. The mass had also grown. I did ask about a prognosis. He said it is very difficult to assess due to Mom having such an atypical cancer. He said she might make it a year, I felt he was being very generous, or she could obstruct tomorrow and that would certainly accelerate things. The good news is that I think that this regimen of pain medication is working. She continues to be positive and have a sense of humor. I thank you for all your prayers. Sue

AUGUST 12, 2001

Mom had a somewhat restless night. She was up five times to go to the bathroom. I still would call it a fair night. She is not waking because of pain and that is good. We did have one episode of losing personal property during the night. We were returning from the bathroom and she asked me if I knew what happened to her panties. She swears she had them on when she went to bed and now they are gone. It was a mystery to me. Then and now.

Around 6:15, she thought some toast would be good, and we chatted while I toasted. She does seem much clearer in her conversation and steadier in her walking. When we walked through the garden, I wish you could have been there. The Beauty Berries are turning purple, and the Brazilian Rock Roses take your breath away. We even pulled a few weeds. "I Come to the Garden Alone" seems to take on a much deeper meaning.

She is asking questions like why they are suggesting that she not start radiation for her throat. I told her that it was suggested last Tuesday, when she was so sick. I also told her that if she wanted radiation she certainly could have radiation. Nobody was parking her in the corner and draping a dropcloth over her. She smiled in response to my comment. She is

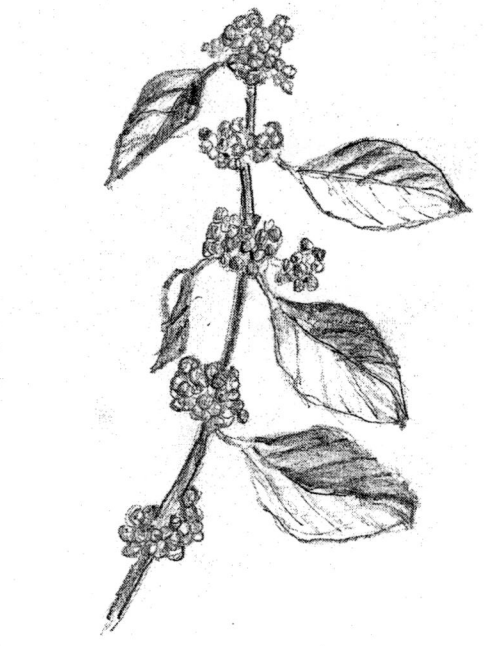

beauty berry

napping right now. I am thinking about taking an inventory of all personal belongings that she was wearing at bedtime in case of a pop quiz. Love, Sue

AUGUST 13, 2001

Mom kind of dozed through the day yesterday. I did a personal inventory around 8:30 p.m. Mom and I both laughed about this. She became restless around 9:30 p.m. I had been asking all day if she felt like she needed a second patch. Dr. C. had said she might need one on Sunday. When asked if she needed it, she said maybe later. She became very restless around midnight and wanted an Ambien. She took it and we both went back to bed. She woke me at two and said she could not stand the pain. I put on another patch and gave her two oxycontin. I told her I was going to be more insistent in the future about her pain medicine.

She woke me again at 3:45 a.m. She was still hurting and said she needed an Immodium because she had been up several times to the bathroom. I gave her two more oxycontins. I checked on her at 5 and she was sleeping. She appeared to be asleep until about 7:30 a.m. when she got up to go to the bathroom.

It was not a good night for her but, maybe she will have a better day. I fertilized all the patio plants at 6:30 a.m. They are beautiful. I will keep you updated. Love, Sue

AUGUST 14, 2001

Becky is Sally's daughter.
Sue has given Sally an old-fashioned bicycle horn to honk
if she needs help in the night.

Mom's afternoon seemed to level off. She told me that she didn't think she could handle another day like Monday again. She and Lynda have conspired to exclude me from cleaning out the freezer today. She is hoping to have enough energy.

Becky is coming to lunch with Mom today. We turned in fairly early. I did a personal inventory. She was going to take the whole Ambien at bedtime. I made her promise me that she would honk for me with the Harpo Marx horn I gave her. I was concerned about the extra sedation. I awoke at 3:30 a.m. and found her cleaning her toilet. She had a close call of the number 2 kind. I fussed at her for not waking me. She said she didn't have time. This will be discussed further in the a.m. She said she wanted another Ambien. She didn't have to wake up early and she wanted to catch up on her sleep. I heard her in the bathroom around 4:45 a.m. I decided to listen for any problems and add this trip to the bathroom to the discussion this morning.

She was asleep by 5 and it is 6:45 now and she is still sleeping. I'm going to start watering and will let you know how the meeting of the minds go. Love, Sue

AUGUST 15, 2001

Well, I think she had a better night. She was up at 2:30, 4:30 and 5:30. There were no traumatic trips to the bathroom. In fact, instead of a bloody discharge, she reported mucus. Just maybe, it has scabbed over or something to that effect. She is more comfortable than she has been in the last couple of days.

The doctor has increased her medication. Her pain lollipops have been increased to 60 mcg and her pain patches (like nicotine patches but deliver pain medicine instead of nicotine) increased 150 mg. I'm not very happy with the doctor. I called yesterday afternoon about Mom bleeding. It was gushing like a very, very heavy period. The floor and her gown needed to be cleaned. My understanding was that I would get a call back. Well, I am still waiting. I'm going to call the doctor this morning, and see if he will order a CBC and if needed, a blood transfusion.

It was hard yesterday. Mom started crying about how extremely tired she was and I became tearful. I promised her that I would get her to feel better and would speak to the doctors about options. I haven't told her yet, but I have talked to the Visiting Nurse Association (Hospice). I think they will do a very good job, the only snag is that they rarely do blood transfusions. I need to scoot now in finish my watering. Love, Sue

AUGUST 18, 2001
Becky, Bryant and Diane are Sally's other children.
Sara and Jacob are her grandchildren.

Mom said she was happy to be able to talk about things so she didn't feel all alone. We made a pact to talk, so none of us had to feel alone. She said that she wasn't afraid of death, she was worried about us. I asked her how she thought we would behave after her funeral. She said Becky would probably vacuum and take care of the food. Bryant would be watching after Jacob and Sara, making sure they knew all the relatives, and Diane and I would be telling funny stories. She said that she felt at peace, seeing me take over the household. She knows, of course, that my health might change, but I would find a way. She said how much she loved all of us and treasured how unique we all were. It was a time of real intimacy. I hope you all get a chance to talk with Mom. She had an outstanding night and is eating toast right now. I love you, Sue

AUGUST 19, 2001

Yesterday Mom had two rough times. The first one, she became tearful and put her head on my shoulder. She said that she didn't think she could handle the pain. I promised to make sure that she would not have to face that question every day. We were close to getting good pain coverage. What we needed to focus on right now is how she felt right now. The pain subsided. I think her extreme fatigue plays the big part in all this. It totally depletes her to walk to the bathroom. She also expressed concern that she didn't want Becky to see her hurt like this. I asked her what her fear was all about. She said Becky tries to put on a brave and cheerful front. I encouraged her to ask Becky how she felt when she saw her in pain. In fact, while I was gone Becky helped Mom through an episode of nausea and did great. Mom did not ask her how she felt about seeing her sick. When I got home, Mom was in good spirits, and she said she was hungry! Becky and Tom had grilled some steaks that morning for Mom. She licked her plate clean. I could have sworn that I heard her chuckle like Jenny does when she's eating Mom's corn pudding. We have talked about playing beauty parlor again. How trusting she is!

Again Mom didn't wake me during the night. She is still asleep so I can't ask her, but I suspect she got up once or twice, but I would bet she had a real good night.

We will have our Sunday brunch today. I usually fix a fancy omelet and the works. She is hoping to put on regular clothes today, a first step to getting her strength back. A second step would be getting a blood transfusion.

We would be lost without the help of Becky and Tom. Becky really freshened up the house and Mom as well. She also bought some pretty sheets and two beautiful gowns. They both have such a wonderful way of knowing what would put a smile on Mom's face. Tom labored over Mom's bed. Before if you sat on the end of the bed, it would come apart. Now I can sit there without tipping Mom out onto the floor. Becky had done the majority of the grocery shopping and Tom worked out in the yard some. I feel so blessed that we can all come together and create a wonderful secure environment for Mom. I know it means a lot to Mom to see her children do what they do the best. I'm going to check on Mom. I will write later. Love, Sue

AUGUST 20, 2001

Yesterday was wonderful. Mom tried out three new recipes. Later we, and I say that loosely, painted fingernails and toenails. With beautiful precision Mom painted her fingernails. She got tickled at me, because as I labored over her toenails…well…because of the position of my head, and my total and complete concentration, I tended to drool. I don't think I inspired much confidence. I just need to practice keeping my mouth closed and swallowing.

We talked about which hospice to go with. She wants to leave that decision to us. We also talked about the blood transfusion. I think she will go along with this. We also talked about the radiation on her throat. I told her it was totally up to her. Mom was Mom yesterday. What a gift.

I assume she slept well. She didn't honk during the night and is still asleep. Well, it is time for me to start the watering of the flowers. I am hoping that Mom can look at her garden today. Love, Sue

Corn Pudding

1 can cream style corn
1 can whole kerrnel corn
½ cup cornbread mix
2 eggs
4 Tbs sugar
1 stick margarine
    Melt margarine in a pyrex dish
    Add drained corn and cornbread mix
    Beat eggs slightly and add to other ingredients
    Bake at 350° for 30 to 40 minutes or until set

AUGUST 20, 2001

Well, Mom just got up and told me that she had been up six times during the night to go to the bathroom. She had also lost her pain sucker and didn't want to wake me up. She asked me to make it all go away, and we both became tearful. I gave her Immodium, a new sucker and two oxycontin capsules. I told her I could sit right there by her till it went away. We will have a talk later about the proper use of her Harpo Marx horn. Love, Sue

AUGUST 21, 2001

Mom had a pretty good day yesterday. The nurse and her tech came to help Mom with her bath. I talked to Becky about my frustration with Mom not using her horn during the night. Becky immediately had a solution. We will get her a little spider monkey. The monkey could help Mom find certain personal belongings, help with grooming, honk her horn and come get me if she tries to get up by herself. Becky is a problem solver. I presented this to Mom with the added problem, I don't do diapers. When being presented with the horn or the monkey, the horn wins hands down.

Her pain patch was changed from 150 to 200mcgs. I hope this is the right dosage. Because we have to consider the morphine pump which Mom doesn't want, her suckers were changed from 600 to 800mcgs. The next strength is 1200mcgs and that is as high as they go. Bryant took the prescription to the pharmacy for Mom. They will deliver it in the morning. Mom's appetite is really back. She completely cleaned her plate. Mom woke me at 12:30 to get her some chips and salsa. She said that previously, she honked and came in and tapped me on the shoulder. I have trouble believing that. I think I would for sure have awakened. Later when Mom got up in the morning she said she had been up a total of four times, and only been able to wake me once. Actually, I think she is really wanting that monkey.

We went out to the garden for a walk. The flowers put on such a show for her. I am waiting to hear from Dr. L. about his suggestion about radiation. Mom goes to see the oncologist on the 24th. Hopefully, he will schedule a blood transfusion. She sees the doctor on the

31st to check on the status of the mass. I am going to close now and go water Mom's flowers. Love, Sue

AUGUST 21, 2001

For the first time in over three weeks, Mom put her yard clothes on and was able to work on her flowers for 30 minutes. I took pictures of this great event. Love, Sue

AUGUST 22, 2001

Mom asked me to look at her sacral area. She complained of a tingling and burning. The area is dark red. She has developed a stage one pressure sore. I put grandmother's sheepskin underneath her. I told her I was going to set my alarm and make sure she is turning from side to side. They recommended an increase in vitamin C, iron and zinc. I am going to check into foam mattress pads. This concerns me because if the skin breaks down in that area, there is a risk of fecal contamination. I spoke to Becky and was taking a more laid-back attitude, but when all cylinders started clicking, I realize we need to treat this very aggressively. Love, Sue

AUGUST 22, 2001

Mom had a great day yesterday. She was able to work in her garden twice. The first time for 30 minutes and the second time for 15 minutes. When she would come into the house, she would stop at the table and close her eyes and whisper the words "Thank you, God." Her appetite is off the charts! She's going through bag of Frito Scoops and Pace extra mild salsa in about a day and a half. She does not even make it two days. In fact, when I went to check on her this morning she was eating Fritos and salsa. She then asked me to make some toast, so she could cleanse her palette. She was already dressed in her yard clothes. She did have a pretty good night. When we were talking this morning, she said she felt like she was climbing out of the hole. I find myself smiling when I think of the nurse tech having to dig Mother out of her garden so she could assist her with a bath. No telling what will happen with Mom charged up on her Frito Scoops and salsa. I will let you know the outcome.

Thank you God, for this day, my Mother and Frito's. Love, Sue

AUGUST 23, 2001
Grace Elizabeth is Sue's chubby, brown dog

Mom spent maybe a total of an hour outside pruning her flowers and complementing them on their style and grace. Bryant was able to be with Mom and follow her directions on what needed to be trimmed, edged or rearranged. The garden is simply beautiful. What a gift from God. Mother is so happy and at peace when she is in her garden.

We had another special treat. Becky and Tom bought Mom one of those wonderful recliners that can lift you to a standing position. They were thinking of the future and how independent Mom is. I have been pleasantly surprised with how Mom is asking for things that she needs and wants. She had a couple of small rough times with nausea, but it subsided fairly quickly. The Chinese barking spiders (gas) were a lot quieter today. They didn't even have their claws out, which really cuts down on the pain.

Mom said she had a pretty good night. There was evidence of Fritos and salsa consumption. I set my alarm and got up several times during the night to check on Mom's position. The stage one pressure sore on her sacral area is still there. The skin is not broken, but the skin is a deep red and does not blanch when pressure is applied. She also complains of tingling and burning. I put grandmother's sheepskin under her and will start some vitamin C, zinc and iron. They are supposed to be helpful. I am becoming more organized than ever before.

While hand watering the flowers on the patio this morning, I used the hose to floss and stimulate Grace's gums. Actually, she didn't give me much choice.

Mom sees her doctor tomorrow and I will let all of you know his recommendations. I will close for now, so I can finish watering the garden.

Thank you God, for this day so sweet, our mother, family and friends and the beauty of your flowers. Love, Sue

AUGUST 24, 2001

Linda is a friend of Sue's

Mom had a busy day yesterday. Andrew came calling. He is Linda's great-grandson and the most beautiful baby. Not to mention personality, plus eight teeth. You couldn't ask for much more, but he has wonderful fashion sense. Mom really enjoyed his visit. The nurse and nurse tech also came. Mom does not really like the tech. Mom says she is too pushy. I think it is a good sign that Mom isn't going to let anyone push her around. I know for a fact that this tech's days are numbered.

Mom hit a few rough times yesterday. The pain really began to increase at bedtime. Things always seem worse at night. I increased her meds and she held my hand and asked me not to leave. As if I would! I told her this is what I was talking about when I told her we don't have to be alone ever. Gracie started to fret; she knew Mom was having a rough time. Mom and I talked about what a good night nurse Grace is. Mom's night was somewhat restless. I think she is also anxious about her doctor's appointment this afternoon. I will let you know what he has to say. I need to finish watering the garden.

Thank you for this day so sweet and baby named Andrew, holding hands with my mother and the night nurse named Grace. Love, Sue

AUGUST 25, 2001

Mom had a pretty rough day yesterday. She was vomiting and in a lot of pain. She was unable to keep her appointment with Dr. W. because of this. I was able to reschedule the appointment for 2:40 Monday. This might work out better because Diane will be here and get a chance to meet her doctor.

Mom got to feeling better around 2:30 and started clipping coupons. She is hoping that someday soon she will be able to go to the store. How she loves to shop and if it is a bargain, it is even more fun. We watched *America's Funniest Videos* and had several big belly laughs. Laughter is truly healing. Mom slept pretty good last night, with only a few trips to the bathroom. After eating her toast this morning, we went out and did some pruning on her flowers. I have bug bites all over my legs. I sure hope they don't turn into Old Testament running sores. They have in the past. Mom did not seem to be bothered by them. She has plans of trying to make a banana pie later.

Thank you God, for this day so sweet, for flowers to be pruned, the healing power of shared laughter and Benadryl cream. Love, Sue

AUGUST 26, 2001
Diane is Sally's oldest daughter

Mom had a much better day yesterday. She just had a few semi-rough times. They passed quickly. She decided to bake some pies yesterday. Yes, pies as in plural. She was restless and when that happens, she cooks in quantity. She sat on her red kitchen stool and commenced to baking. When she finished, we had a coconut- banana pie and a strawberry cream pie with a semisweet chocolate coating on the crust.

Becky and Tom came to see Mom. Becky had a satin pillowcase to protect Mom's hairdo. Becky fixes Mom's hair every Saturday. Mom does have a beautiful full head of white hair. Our neighbor, Lisa , came over in the afternoon to fertilize Mom's flowers. It is a real blessing to have such good neighbors.

Mom had a real big surprise when Diane walked into her room at 7:30 last night. Her baby was in her room and she could not have been happier. I was beside myself that my older sister was here. I had prayed that Diane would be able to come and spend time with Mom before it was too late. None of us knows what tomorrow brings. This is certainly not the time to postpone anything you want to say or do. Mom fell asleep to the sound of her daughters laughing and telling stories.

Mom just got up and I made her morning toast for her. She said she had a pretty peaceful night knowing that her oldest child was asleep in the next room.

Thank you God for this day so sweet, wondrous smells from the kitchen, good neighbors and for the gift of Diane's visit. Well, it is time to start my watering. Love, Sue

AUGUST 28, 2001

We made it to see the on-cologist yesterday afternoon. He was very kind and a very good listener. He proposed several options, the first being that she could go see a gynecological on-cologist, and he might be able to get a biopsy. With a biopsy they could then do radiation and at least reduce the size of the tumor. There are potential negative side effects. Mom also could choose to go into hospice for more sup-portive care. Her primary con-cern was good pain control. He made the comment that her blood work had improved and if she wanted a blood transfusion he would order it. She became a little tearful; she said that she was hurting and feeling overwhelmed

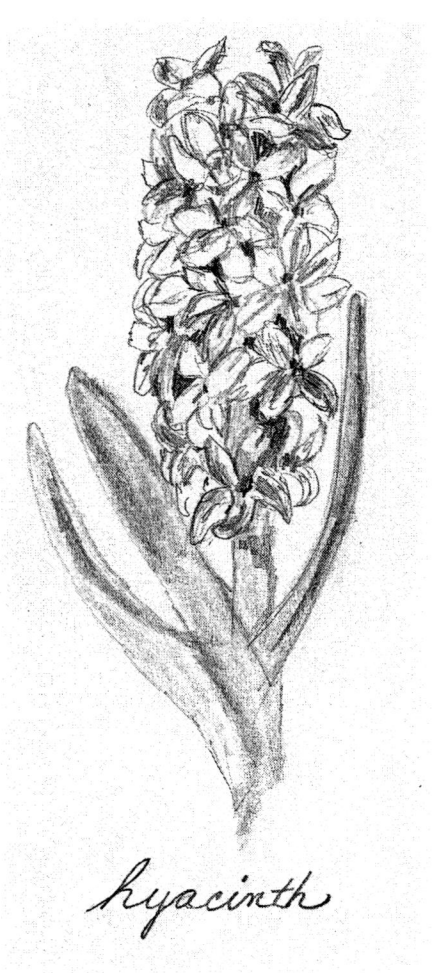

hyacinth

and wanted to take some time to make a decision. We are calling him with her decision.

We made our way home, but stopped to get Mom some onion rings and Diane and me a coconut cream pie shake. The car was full of a lot of contented food sounds. After dinner, Diane crawled into bed with Mom. It did not take long for both of them to move into taking a power nap. At 9:00 I turned out the lights and Grace and I went to bed. It had been a very long day.

I got up at six this morning and went to check on Mom. She had a rough night with many trips to the bathroom. Of course, she had not used the horn. I see a monkey looming in Mom's future. Maybe I could do a motion detector at her door that would alert me. I will think about that later.

Mom had wanted her toast with pear preserves and cantaloupe. While she was eating her toast, we began to talk. Mom expressed concern that we would think she was a chicken if she chose hospice. She also voiced concerns about being isolated from people because of their discomfort with the subject of dying. I told Mom that she could never disappoint us. She was not giving up because she was choosing hospice. There is a whole lot of living that goes on in hospice. That was my experience when I worked in hospice. It seems that life becomes more focused and sweeter. You begin to live as we all should live, in the here and now. I told her that she had the comfort and peace of our faith in God and was surrounded with family and friends that loved her and wanted to be included in her life. Diane woke up and joined our talk. I left the room to give them some private time. I later asked Diane if she could water the container plants and Mom popped up and said "Let's do it together!"

I will shortly be calling the doctor so he can make the referral to hospice.

Thank you God for this day so sweet, for doctors who listen, onion rings, morning talks with Mom and for your peace that fills our hearts and home. Love, Sue

AUGUST 29, 2001

Mom had kind of an up-and-down day. She had more trouble with nausea. Hospice received the order from the doctor to admit Mom to their program. A nurse will come today to fill out all the paperwork and answer any questions that we might have. Mom seemed to withdraw a little when I told her that hospice would start tomorrow. She denied feeling overwhelmed but this was a big decision. She is afraid that people will perceive her as being chicken. I will print any messages that any of you might want to send to Mom. I have reassured her that we were are all here for her. Diane and I have both told her that hospice is a choice and is absolutely about quality-of-life.

Yesterday Diane volunteered to water the patio plants and asked me how much watering the plants needed. Mom popped up and said "Let's do it together!" This was such a tender moment with Diane and Mom. It has been a help having Diane here. I stayed home and prepared dinner and Diane went and ran errands for Mom. Becky was at her office, but was dealing with all that goes with trying to get insurance to pay. Bryant came over and brought Sara for a visit. I pray Mom feels our love as we all gather around her.

I checked on Mom around 2 a.m. She was sleeping hard. I smiled when I saw the Fritos and salsa by her bed. She says she slept well last night. She does appear more relaxed this morning. Diane was awake and participated in the ritual of morning talk and toast.

Thank you God for this day so sweet, the comfort of a peaceful sleep and for morning talks and toast. Love, Sue

AUGUST 30, 2001

Mom's first day of hospice was yesterday. The admitting nurse's name was Anna. She was wonderful and a very good listener. It is a very involved process with all the paperwork that they have to do. Mom will have to switch doctors. Mom was pleased that she had the opportunity to see all of her children yesterday. Bryant dropped by twice and Becky came on her lunch break bearing bowls of wonderful soup. Mom is a big fan of all kinds of soup. We were both very pleased when we saw what a wonderful job our new yard man had done. He trimmed hedges and cleaned out flower beds. Mom's garden continues to be a thing of beauty.

Mom had a few rough times yesterday. We are still trying to fine tune her pain medicine. I had prepared a roast, fresh green beans and mashed potatoes for dinner and Mom was able to sit at the table for the first time in weeks. For the most part, Mom had a pretty good night. I had set my alarm for 1 a.m. so I could make sure she got her dose of oxycontin. She was awake and seemed relieved to see me. I reset my alarm for 5:30 so I could check to see if she needed another dose. Diane happened to awake at 5 and woke me because she needed the oxycontin for Mom. I am so glad that Diane is here.

I went to check on Mom at 6 and she was getting out of bed. I started to tell her good morning, when she held her finger to her lips and pointed to Diane and the bed. It was such a tender moment for me. Mother is still Mother. It is raining here this morning. Mom sat on the porch and enjoyed the rain and watched as morning arrived. Mom and Diane had their talk and toast this morning at the breakfast table.

Thank you God, for this day so sweet, a nurse named Anna, heart-warming bowls of soup and morning rain. Love, Sue

AUGUST 31, 2001

Mom had a stressful morning. She has complained at various times of epigastric fullness. This is probably a hiatal hernia. With the fullness, at times, she has also experienced shortness of breath. In addition to the symptoms, she began coughing and coughing. I had an extra oxygen tank, so I started her on some oxygen and found her nebulizer and medication. After two treatments her coughing eased and she was not complaining of not being able to catch her breath. I certainly know how scary that can feel. I contacted hospice and they are sending out a concentrator in case she has any other episodes of shortness of breath. The concentrator provides her oxygen.

The hospice social worker came out to talk with us. Mom was too tired to talk, so she spoke to Diane and me. She was reviewing the different levels of care that hospice offers. We discussed my health and what might happen if I at some point am not able to meet Mom's changing needs. I told her that God has blessed me thus far with the energy to provide care for Mom and the house. This is truly a blessing because I don't know where it comes from. I told her that we had a good network of family and friends to help. Lynda, a friend of mine, has made the commitment to help in any way necessary to provide the comfort and support to Mom. We also have the most wonderfully involved neighbors. Diane and I told her that we were prepared to do whatever it took to keep Mom in her home and in her bed...the bed that she was born in. It seems so fitting that she will end her life in the bed where she was given life. The social worker will also be sending out a chaplain to talk with Mom, and she also thought she could find a volunteer to help with watering the flowers.

Yesterday the rain stayed with us all day, which made for good sleeping weather. I guess you might see where I'm going with this. Mom and Diane took a very long nap and I finished reading a book called *Peaceful Dying*. It is written by a doctor who has a terminal illness. It was a day filled with quiet talks interrupted with some deep soul satisfying laughter. Bryant and the kids came over for a visit with Mom. They are really growing up.

I went to bed early and Diane stayed up to help Mom with her medicine and to properly tuck her in for the night. I awoke at 5 to check to see if Mom needed her medicine. She's sleeping so soundly that I decided not to wake her at this time. I put on an Elvis Presley gospel CD and decided to write the morning note. This is a wonderful time of the morning.

Thank you God, for this day so sweet, the healing power of laughter and your music that brings such peace and comfort. Love, Sue

SEPTEMBER 1, 2001

Becky is Sally's youngest daughter.
Tom is Becky's husband and Sherri is their daughter.
Uncle William is Sally's older brother. Aunt MM is his wife.
Bryant is Sally's son. Sara and Jacob are his children.

Mom had a full afternoon yesterday. She met with Janet, the chaplain, and Laurie, the nurse. Janet was very easy to talk with. At one point in the conversation Diane got up and left the room. Janet suggested that we all share a prayer so I went to get Diane. I found her in the bathroom sobbing. She initially said that she could not come because she was not in control. She responded to my encouragement that she not hide her tears from Mom. She climbed into bed with Mom and expressed her fears about living in a world where she could not reach out and touch her mother. Mom reminded her that she would always be in her heart. It was a powerful moment between Diane and Mom. Diane and Mom spent the rest of the day going through old papers, old pictures and recipes to clean out some of the clutter from her room. Laurie had observed that Mom was running a slight temperature. I don't know if the source is bladder or lungs. She has been wheezing. Diane volunteered to give Mom her oxycontin around 1 a.m. to keep the pain in check.

This morning, when she woke me she told me that Mom had an extremely restless night. She seemed to be in constant motion in her sleep. At one point Diane found her preparing a major fruit salad in the kitchen. Diane decided to sleep with Mom, so she would be right there if Mom should need her. I pray that we are not going to go through another episode of altered mental status. When I went to check on Mom, I gave her some toast and an aspirin. She was pretty cranky. She is mentally clear this morning.

It is raining here, and Mom and I took a walk to the front porch to get a change in scenery. A neighbor came up to visit for moment. This is going to be a busy day. Becky, Tom and Sherri are coming at noon. Becky will do Mom's hair and hopefully have a good visit. Tom and Sherri will also visit, but will look to see if there are any chores that need to be done. Uncle William and Aunt MM are also going to stop by for a short visit. Bryant said he would come by later with Jacob and Sara. The kids are so tender with Mom. Right now Diane is asleep in my bed, Mom is in her bed reading the new Southern Living magazine and Grace Elizabeth is guarding her food bowl.

Thank you God, for this day so sweet, the much needed rain and the healing power of shared tears. Love, Sue

SEPTEMBER 2, 2001.
Gordon, Diane's husband is very ill. Jenny is Diane's daughter.

Yesterday was a nice day. We all had breakfast together. I had fixed ham and eggs and toast. Mom accused me of giving her a dozen eggs to eat. She did clean her plate. Becky, Tom and Sherri came for a visit. Tom put up a new grab bar by Mom's tub. Becky brought homemade potato soup with all the fixin's and her famous brownies. Her brownies are like crack. Once you have tasted them, you lose all rational thought about portion control. Diane had to double up on her pepcid. My conscience is clear; I did try to warn her. Sherri visited with Mom and worked on a paper for school. Becky also helped Mom to freshen up. When Becky freshens, it is not with just a moist towelette. She does such a wonderful job on Mom's hair. It has kind of been a laid-back Saturday. I am not looking forward to Sunday. Diane has to go back to Beaumont. It has been very comforting to have someone to share, not just the daily chores, but the emotions that catch you off-guard. I know that Diane faces the larger challenge of having to say goodbye to Mom today. She will be back to see Mom, but you never know if this is going to be your last goodbye.

I am touched by Jenny's generosity in stepping up and taking on the demands of caring for her father, while trying to get her semester at college off to a start. Diane was able to let go of worrying about the ongoing care of Gordon and truly be there for her mother. None of us knows how long we have. Diane really spent her time well with Mom talking, laughing, crying, nurturing and caring for Mom and allowing Mom to mother her. I really consider myself so blessed to be here with Mom. God will provide what is needed to care for her. Mom had a pretty restless night. She had taken an extra dose of Milk of Magnesia and you can figure out the implications of that action. She did not wake me. I had set my alarm for 2 a.m. to see if she was hurting and needed her oxycontin. She said she was fine. I did hear her in the bathroom at 5 a.m. I usually awake at 5 a.m. to have a quiet time before my day starts. Diane got up at 7 a.m. and visited with Mom for a while. They both decided to grab a quick morning nap before the day really got started. Diane came and climbed in my bed while I sit here finishing my morning note. The whole house has a very peaceful feel to it.

Thank you God, for this day so sweet, a niece named Jenny, crack brownies and pepcid. Love, Sue

Becky's Crack Brownies

2 Sticks butter

2 cups sugar

4 eggs

1½ cups flour

6 Tbs cocoa

2 Tbs vanilla

    Set oven at 350° and grease 9 x 13 glass baking dish

    Blend butter and add eggs 1 at a time

    Add flour, cocoa and vanilla

    Pour into greased baking dish

    Bake 30 minutes

Topping

½ stick butter

2 Tbs cocoa

4 Tbs milk

8 oz. powdered sugar

    Melt butter and stir in rest of ingredients

    Poke holes in top of warm brownies and pour over

SEPTEMBER 5, 2001

Yesterday was a very difficult day for Mom and me. It was as if a dark cloud had moved and settled right over Mom's bed. At first she told me that her left foot felt heavy and numb. She insisted that it was not like it had fallen asleep. Of course, this impacted her walking. She did not want to move without holding on to me, which was fine. Maybe the tumor is pressing on a nerve.

I sat on the end of her bed while she ate her toast. I started seeing tears roll out of the corner of her eyes. I questioned her softly about what might be wrong. She would shake her head and say, "I don't know what is wrong." I told her that she did not have to have a reason for her tears. I also reassured her that her tears were not going to push me away. I did talk about grieving and how her children weren't the only ones grieving. She also was grieving over many things, such as feeling more dependent, feeling like her body had betrayed her, the many recent life changes in this past month. I made myself stay, but the little girl in me wanted to run for help. My Mom was crying and someone needed to make things ok again.

When Uncle William and Aunt MM stopped by for a visit Mom was not able to hide how she felt. Uncle William was so overwhelmed to see Mom like that, he had to cut their visit short. He later called me and said that he was sorry, but he did not want Mom to see him cry. I told him that it was ok to share his tears with Mom.

A new nurse, named Christy, came to check on Mom. Laurie, the nurse that admitted her, had a big caseload and they wanted to be sure that Mom received all the attention that she needed or wanted. Again Mom did not try to hide how blue she felt. We were walking down the hall to the bathroom and I asked her if she wanted to take a detour to see her flowers. She answered with a firm flat out "No!" I later talked with Mom about how sometimes we all need a day when we can pull the covers over our heads. But tomorrow was going to be full when the aide comes to help her with a bath and she goes for a walk to check out her flowers and she helps me plan dinner. We might even get a Skip-Bo game in.

Mom was up three times to the bathroom, but all in all had a fairly restful night. This morning, she got up and washed her face, brushed her teeth and combed her hair. Let's hear it for Mom!

Thank you God for this day so sweet, for the peace that allowed me to stay and not run away from Mother's tears and new beginnings. Love, Sue

SEPTEMBER 10, 2001

Mom had a good day yesterday. Her first words to me yesterday were, "I had a good night's sleep and I don't hurt!" Mother and I broke out into great big smiles. Someone observing this exchange would think we had won the lottery. It was better than the lottery. It was respite from the constant pain. Mom finally had a taste of what it was like to be pain-free. I feel that it gave her hope that she was not sentenced to pain without the possibility of parole. She asked for an omelet for breakfast. While I was preparing breakfast, she sat in the recliner reading the Sunday paper and clipping coupons. We bowed our heads and shared a prayer of gratitude before we had breakfast.

Later Mom enjoyed reading her e-mails that had come in during the morning. The computer has been a real blessing in keeping family and friends connected. Uncle William and Aunt MM came by after church. They were pleasantly surprised to see Mom sitting up and pain-free. Margaret, our neighbor, came by for a surprise visit. She brought the most beautiful lilies from her garden. Towards the end of their visit Mom experienced a bout of nausea. It passed quickly after taking some Compazine. After dinner Bryant and Jacob came by for a visit. At bedtime Mom was glowing about what a wonderful day she had.

When I got up to check on Mom during the night there was evidence of serious snacking. At 5, when I went to check on her, she reported having another good night's sleep, but that she was ready for her pain medication. Just maybe she is learning not to let the pain get out of control before she asks for her medication.

I am so excited! I went to let Grace outside and I was met with cool weather. The first sign that fall and winter are on the way. For all that know me, cold is how I like it. I almost felt like doing a cartwheel. I am sure Grace is pleased that I didn't act on that urge. We have an agreement in place not to participate in any gravity defying acts.

Thank you God, for this day so sweet, for flowers from a good friend's garden, for the changing of the seasons and for the reminder that you are with us always. Love, Sue

SEPTEMBER 11, 2001

Mother had another good day yesterday. She said that she couldn't believe that this was her third good night of sleep. She continues to report that the pain has greatly diminished. We had our usual toast and talk. She spoke of how much it means to her to get these daily e-mails from Jenny and Diane. It feels almost like they have joined us for toast. After breakfast Mom decided to take a tour of her garden. She saw some things that needed pruning and took care of it with the precision of a surgeon. Shortly after we went back into the house her nurse, Christy, arrived. She seemed pleased that Mom's pain had decreased. We discussed again the possibility of changing from the patches to an oral medication. Evidently the patches really aren't very effective on folks who weigh less than 100 lbs. She brought her scale to weigh Mom. Her scale read 90 lbs., but I believe Mom probably weighs closer to 95. I will have Mom weigh on the doctor's scale to compare her reading. We talked again about Mom taking elavil. I expressed my concern about Mom experiencing orthostatic hypotension. If I can get Mom's solemn promise that she will not move out of bed without double honking for me, I will give it a try. Tuesday night everybody please say a prayer for Mom that she will use her horn with great vigor to wake me up.

Caroline, her aide, came at 3 to help with her bath. She also put fresh sheets on the bed. She is tall and has a ready smile. Mother took her outside to share her garden with her. I think she is really beginning to bond with her. Mom started having really sharp gas pains. Basically all you can do is wait for it to subside. I did give her a pill around 5 p.m., which helps with spasms in the bowel. She appeared to get some relief and fell asleep. She slept until 7:30. She wasn't very hungry and will probably snack later.

Mother and I are going to set aside time tonight, right before bed to say our prayers. Together, we said The Lord's Prayer and I Lay Me Down to Sleep. Mom and I talked about saying our prayers, not only at night, but in the morning and any other time that comes up during the day.

Mom and I turned in at our usual time, 9:00 p.m. She was awake three times during the night. The horn was given a workout each time. Mom says that she would count this as a restful night. When I opened the door to let Grace out I was met with even cooler temperatures. My heart started racing. I was so excited. I told Mom that I was fighting back the impulse to go out and roll in the grass. You would think Mom would have looked at me strangely, but she smiled and patted me on the hand and said, "You really get so happy when the cool temperatures move in." Grace came in later bragging that, not only had she taken a roll in the grass, she had found something wonderful to roll in. There is a difference between us. I would not have bragged.

Thank you God, for this day so sweet, the smell of fresh sheets, the gift of prayer and having a mother who not only knows, but loves even the peculiar aspects of our personalities. Love, Sue

SEPTEMBER 12, 2001.
FiFi is Sally's older sister. Linc is Sally's close friend

Mom had one rough patch yesterday. Unfortunately, we had to cancel her appointment with the doctor. It will be rescheduled for next Tuesday. We both spent the morning watching TV coverage on the attacks on New York. Debi called her mother to let her know she was safe. Like so many others that had lived through Pearl Harbor, Mom said that she never expected to see anything like that again in her lifetime. Lynda came by carrying a fresh loaf of salt risen bread and news about how big Andrew is getting. Mom surprised us both by challenging us to a game of Skip-Bo. She even played it at the kitchen table. I surprised us all by winning the game. She even surprised me more when she asked me for some Fritos and salsa. She had this little grin on her face when she said, "I am still full of surprises!" These words warmed me through and through. I said a prayer of gratitude.

Aunt FiFi called and they both reflected on where they were when they heard the news of Pearl Harbor. How blessed Mom is to have an older sister, not to mention what a wonderful and attentive older brother she has. It is humbling to think of all they have lived through and how their faith continues to sustain them. The same faith will sustain them as they say goodbye to their baby sister.

Lynda went to a restaurant and brought back wonderful barbecued ribs and beef. Mom had been craving some good barbecue. As we were beginning to wind up the day Mom called Linc and Bryant to make sure that they were ok. Mom was able to reassure me that she would honk most vigorously if she needed me. She also promised that she would not move from the bed without my help. I am so very cautious about adding new medications. Mom woke me three times during the night to go to the bathroom and to take her oxycontin. She was a little unsteady as she walked. I praised her for honking.

When Mom honks it sets off a chain reaction. Grace barks to let

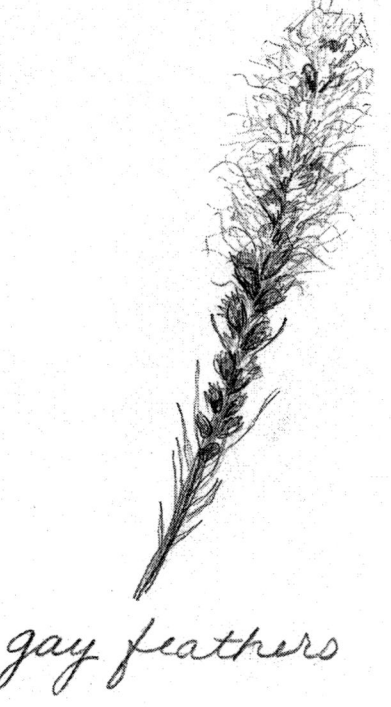

gay feathers

her know she is on the way and I call "I am coming, Mom!" Then the parade begins down the hall. The cats will join in on occasion, only if they feel like they can add some class to the parade. Most of the time Grace leads the way. Frequently Mom and I feel like we got behind a very slow moving truck hauling logs and we are in a no pass lane. It is times like these when you are reacquainted with the virtue of patience. We also said our prayers together. I am so glad that this has become a part of our bedtime ritual.

Thank you God, for this day so sweet, for the gift of having older siblings and the memories they share and for the wonder of parades, no matter how small they might be. Love, Sue

SEPTEMBER 14, 2001

Marilyn is a former co-worker of Sally's

Mom had a sleepy day yesterday. I think there is a hangover effect from the elavil. Janet, the hospice chaplain, came by for a visit. At one point, Mom was in the bathroom and Janet said she had a hard question to ask me. I braced myself and realized that she was talking about Mom's DNR (do not resuscitate) status. I told her that we just needed to get Mom and the doctor to sign it. I also told her when they gave it to me to be signed, Mom was short of breath. I would not want anybody talking to me about DNR if I were short of breath. This form actually protects Mom at home if 911 should happen to get called. She has said that she does not want any heroics.

Bryant came over to stay with Mom while I ran to the store. He had a chance to meet Janet. When I returned from the store Reverend Bennett and his wife were here. They were only here for short while. I am sure they could tell how tired she was. After everybody left, I was able to lay down for about half an hour and get my wind back.

Mom and I were pleasantly surprised when Marilyn came by with a wonderful chicken casserole and a card with signatures from all the retired teachers from their luncheon and also a picture of all of them. Mom has the best friends. Of course, Mom taught us in order to have a good friend you need to be a good friend and how true those words ring today. Mom also taught us about "please" and "thank you" and don't take the last piece of anything and what goes around comes around and remember to say your prayers.

The remainder of the evening came to a quiet close when we said our evening prayers. Mom was up several times during the night, but it was a much more restful night. In fact, I hopped up several times only to find out I had dreamed hearing her honk. I am sure it was a dream, only because the cats don't have thumbs to honk with. They have a strange sense of humor and I'm sure they enjoyed watching Grace and me run up the hall to find a sleeping mother. I do know for a fact that Ringo removed the top to the canister of brown sugar. All I know is, you can ask a cat why, and he will laugh in your face. Anyway it was a better night than last night.

Thank you God, for this day so sweet, lessons learned at your mother's knee and the mystery of cats. Love, Sue

SEPTEMBER 15, 2001

Mom slept most of the day yesterday. Her nurse Christy came around 10 to check on her. There were no medication changes. Mom said she was hungry so I scrambled two eggs and cooked some bacon. Mom only ate half of her breakfast. I read the e-mails to her that Jenny and Diane had sent. This is always a favorite part of her day. She fell asleep soon afterwards. Carolyn, her aide, came at 3 p.m. to help her with her bath and change her sheets. Mom said she wanted to talk to me after Carolyn left.

I sat on the end of her bed as she struggled to find her words. She said that she was concerned about how much time today was spent asleep. Tears rolled down her cheeks as she spoke of how she did not want to sleep her days away. She said that she was not hurting, but she could not stay awake. I told her that we could make some changes in her medication. I also suggested that we get some blood work to check on her thyroid. I mainly sat and held her hand while she cried, a seemingly simple, but very difficult task…not to fill up the silence with anxious words.

UPS finally brought the special temperpedic mattress and pillow for Mom. I will wait for Becky's help to get the mattress on the bed. Mom says the pillow feels wonderful. Lisa, our next door neighbor, called to tell us she had made extra spaghetti and meatballs and would like to bring a bowl over for our dinner. Mother and I talked about what good neighbors Lisa and Joe are to us.

I finished watering outdoors and came in and we talked about a fall garden. Mom and I watched a show on antiques, said our prayers and turned in for the night. Mom did not call me during the night. When I got up to check on her I had to smile when I found Fritos and salsa. She says this morning that she had a restful pain-free night.

Thank you God, for this day so sweet, a good neighbor's homemade spaghetti and for heart-to-heart talks with my mother. Love, Sue

SEPTEMBER 17, 2001

Yesterday was a good day for Mom. She was surprised by a visit from her sister FiFi, Uncle Dade and their son Stephen. Stephen flew in from Detroit last night and plans to spend a week in Denton visiting his parents. What a gift for him to get up and drive his folks to Dallas to see Mom. Uncle William and Aunt MM also came by for a visit. They all had a chance for "remember when" stories. They also had an opportunity for shared tears. Aunt FiFi seemed touched when I told her how much Mom enjoyed her daily notes in the mail and how she was the reason Diane and Jenny started writing daily e-mail notes. I made sure that I got pictures of all three of them together. The visit was soon over and the goodbyes I am sure were particularly hard for Aunt FiFi. She can only come when Stephen visits. He is planning on a return visit at the end of October. I'm sure they will be back for a visit at that time.

Mom took a nap while I was preparing a chicken and dumpling dinner. It wasn't like Mom's dumplings, but nothing can compare to your mother's cooking. Lisa and Dria stopped by for a visit and brought Mom some banana nut bread. Bryant came by to see how Mom's Sunday had been. She told him that it had been full of wonderful surprise visits.

Mother honked and said she was ready to be tucked in. Bryant told Mother that he could have helped her. Mother said, "Well, you don't know how Sue arranges the pillows and covers." Bryant and I smiled at each other as I showed him the right way to tuck Mom in. He is now a certified bed-tucker. Bedtime rituals can be such a powerful and comforting act. All of us have bedtime memories, as a child, that comfort us as adults. Bedtime prayers are an important part of our bedtime ritual. They were an important part of my childhood and Mom says prayers were part of her bedtime too.

I was so pleased to hear Mom be so vocal about what felt good to her. Last night was the first time that I realized Mother enjoys the tucking in and saying our prayers as much as I did. I am aware, in the back of my mind, that this might be our last goodnight. She knows that she is loved by her children, but I want her to experience the tenderness and love we have for her.

Mother had a fairly restful night. We were up three times during the night. As I am typing this Mom woke up and let me know that it is time for our morning ritual, talk and toast.

Thank you God for this day so sweet, surprise visits from a loving sister and brother and the peace that comes with prayers at bedtime. Love, Sue

Mother had a fairly good day yesterday. She had only one rough patch with nausea. Her nurse, Christy, came in the morning. We talked some about the possibility of using Ritalin to give her energy a boost. Carolyn, her aide, came in the afternoon. Mom was pleased that her soap operas were back on. Her candle tree now has a third set of blooms. Delbert, (a friend who is a craftsman when it comes to laying brick and stone) came over and we talked about repairing the wall around the patio and taking out the old grill. Mom seemed excited when I told her that I thought he could do it for a song. It would certainly add to the beauty of her beloved garden.

I spent some time working on Max's tail. She is the Persian and had some huge hairballs at the base of her tail. She will let me comb her, but has always considered that area off-limits. She is one of the strongest cats I have ever dealt with. Plus, she must be double-jointed, because she has the ability to unhook her joints and squeeze out of the tightest situations. But I have this special comb and she was somewhat cooperative with me as I tried to remove those awful hairballs. I had also promised her that she would be beautiful after I had finished combing her. Unfortunately things took a turn for the worse. I removed a lot more hair from her tail than I had planned. She looks like she has the "lion tail" you know how the tail appears hairless until you get to the tip of the tail and then there is a tuft of fur. I tried to convince her that she was a trendsetter; pretty soon all the cats would want their tail style that way. Mom just laughed at my trying to explain how I got carried away with playing beauty parlor with Max. Mom and I laughed out loud as Ringo attempted to bathe Max's tail. Max was having no part of this. It felt so good to laugh with Mom.

This evening I prepared a pretty good dinner. Mom sheepishly asked if it would hurt my feelings if she had chips and salsa. I told her "no", I wouldn't be offended. She said she was really experiencing some major cravings for salty things.

Bryant, Jacob and Sara came by for a visit. Mom does enjoy her grandchildren. After they left, I tucked Mom in and we said our prayers. Mom did not honk for me during the night. I did get up to check on her and she had been up to get her Fritos and salsa. She is still sleeping as I write this, so I assume she had a good night. We go to see the doctor at 1:30 this afternoon. I suspect that he will change Mom's pain medicine from patches to oxycontin. I will let you know how it goes.

Thank you God, for this day so sweet, grandchildren and shared laughter. Love, Sue

SEPTEMBER 19, 2001
Kelly is a friend of Sue's

Yesterday was a full day for Mom. We got to the doctor's office before our 1:30 appointment time. The office was full and I knew we had a wait on our hands. I need to mention now that I had not had breakfast or lunch. I knew Mom had toast for breakfast and Lynda said she had not eaten. My stomach began grinding and roaring. It sounded like we had airplanes landing right there in the waiting room. Mom and Lynda were too delicate to make any noise and if they did, it would not sound like fighter jets taking off. Well, 2:30 came and went and 3:30 came and went. Lynda had offered to ask this lady that had a baby with her if she had any extra crackers. I threatened her life if she acted on this idea. I considered ordering a pizza to be delivered, when I thought we had been saved. They said it was our turn. We went into the waiting room and began a new and desperate kind of wait. The sound effects for my stomach had evolved. It sounded like my stomach was speaking in tongues. All of a sudden Mom got up, grabbed her cane and started walking for the door. She opened the door and stepped up to the receptionist desk and asked how much longer she would have to wait. She was tired and did they have any crackers. Well, they had crackers. As Mom turned to come back in the exam room carrying those crackers, she was wearing the biggest catfish grin on her face. I wanted to crawl under my chair. Mom was being Mom. Whatever her children need or want they will have. I ate 3 crackers in a hurry because we were expecting the doctor at any moment. Lynda ate a couple of crackers also, but Mom never touched them. The doctor finally came in and was most apologetic. There had been some emergencies that he had to take care of. It was good to see him.

We talked about Mom's lack of energy and the change to oxycontin from the patch. He suggested that Mom try a low dose steroid which would increase her appetite, increase her energy and also give her a sense of well-being. He also agreed with the suggestion to try her on some low dose Ritalin. These are medications we used when I worked in hospice many years back. Mom has things she wants to do but has been unable to because of no energy and the sedation that comes with the narcotics. He asked if there was anything else he could do for Mom and Mom said, "Yes, there is. You come over here and give me hug." I was so touched with what I saw. The doctor and Mom began their teamwork five years ago.

It was time to go. Mom wanted to take the crackers with us. I told her there was no way I was going take the rest of that lady's crackers. On our way home, we stopped at Jack in the Box and got tacos. I know, but we were desperate. It was after five. When we got home, we were treated to a surprise visit from Kelly. She had rescued some baby birds that were found downtown and had taken them to a wildlife rescue place that would take care of them. That is my kind of friend. Mom headed toward her bed and was asleep before her head hit the pillow. I woke her at 9:30 so she could take her medicine, eat something and change into her gown. I tucked her in and we said our prayers. When I went to check on her I saw where she had gotten up and got her Fritos and salsa. We both slept late this morning.

Thank you God, for this day so sweet, for doctors that hug their patients, emergency crackers and for friends that take the time to rescue baby birds. Love, Sue

SEPTEMBER 20, 2001

Mom had a full day yesterday. Her nurse and aide came by for their routine visit. Lynda and I had made plans to go out to eat and to a show. Bryant, Jacob and Sara came over to stay with Mom while I was gone. As we were leaving, Marilyn arrived carrying a wonderful homemade squash casserole and beautiful stuffed tomatoes. Lynda and I enjoyed the movie. After the movie, we went to El Fenix to eat. I brought home some tortilla soup, chili con queso and fajitas. Mom does love Mexican food. She was so pleased with all her goodies. Bryant and Jacob kissed Mom goodnight and headed home because it was a school night. She had to sample the fajitas and nachos before she went to bed.

Mom was full of stories about all the visitors she had while I was gone. Marilyn was able to stay for a short while and seemed pleased when she found out that Mom was having her ham and bean soup for dinner. Later, Mom's neighbor that lives directly behind her came to check on her. She had become concerned because it had been some time since she had seen Mom working in her alley garden. The neighbor told Mom that her husband had suffered several severe heart attacks and had become extremely dependent on her. She described feeling tied down and trapped. I will explain in the moment why I am writing about her. Then our wonderful neighbor that lives across the street stopped by and brought Mom some coleslaw.

After all her visitors left, Mom and I took a walk in the garden. Mom began apologizing for being such a drain on me. She said that she worried because I did not get out of the house very often. I noticed that she was beginning to tear up. Then, it dawned on me that she had taken to heart what the neighbor had said about feeling trapped and tied down. I asked Mom if she thought I felt like the neighbor. She nodded her head "yes." I took her hand in my hand and said, "I am not the neighbor. I have many people that have volunteered to stay with you if I needed or wanted to get out. I consider it a blessing to have this time to spend with you. I would never use the word burden when talking about how I feel about you. Of all your children, I consider myself luckiest because I share a home with you. I have the chance every day to have morning toast and talk with you and at the end of the day, I get to tuck you in and say our prayers. My life could not be any fuller." Mom was then able to acknowledge that she had probably jumped to the wrong conclusion after listening to the neighbor. I reminded Mom how important it is to check these kinds of feelings out with folks.

After our talk, I tucked Mom in, we said our prayers and turned in for the night. Mom honked for me a couple of times last night. At 1:30 a.m. she asked for her sleeping pill. She is still asleep as I write this note.

Thank you God, for this day so sweet, for fun nights out with my best friend and heart to heart talks with my mother. Love, Sue

SEPTEMBER 22, 2001

Mom had a pretty good day yesterday. Lynda came by, so she could meet Mom's nurse, Christy. Her nurse arrived to do an assessment and was very patient with Mom. Mom was a little spacey from her pain medicine being doubled the night before. After several minutes would seem to pass, I would attempt to answer a question, maybe about her bowel activity. She told me she was capable of answering her own questions and would do so shortly. Well, time passed and nothing was being said soooo…I proceeded to try to help the interview along by answering another question. She told me again that she would answer the questions in her own time. I said, in that case, I had some chores that needed to be done. So Lynda and I left the room.

I was glad that I had Lynda as an independent witness. I know Mom was a little looped, but it looked to me like she was being purposefully difficult. Mom had talked earlier about how she hated answering the same question over and over. I guess she was doing a kind of passive Ghandi protest. After Christy left, Bryant stopped by to give Mom a cane that he had carved. It is beautiful. The hand is carved like a bird head. Then Carolyn, her aide, arrived to help Mom. Lynda left to pick up some groceries for the house. I had an opportunity to sit at the end of Mom's bed and talk with her. I asked Mom if she was feeling depressed. She quickly responded with a "yes", she said she didn't know why. I told her I could think of several things, but I told her that you don't have to have a reason to feel depressed. I told her that Marianne, the social worker, was coming by in a few minutes and could be very helpful in sorting out the feelings she was having. Lynda and Marianne arrived at the same time. Marianne went to talk with Mom and Lynda started frying the cornbread and I folded sheets. After Marianne finished talking with Mom, she came in the kitchen and sat down with us. She had picked up that Mom was headstrong. I asked her if Mom talked very much. She said that Mom did most of the talking. I was very pleased because she needs someone other than her children to talk to. It didn't seem like she would be doing much talking with her nurse. It could not have worked out better. By this time, we were ready for Marilyn's ham and bean soup and Lynda's fried cornbread. Mom really had a feast.

Christy called and said that the doctor had called and was starting Mom on 20 mgs of prednisone twice a day. That is the big dose. In a couple of days Mom will have eaten her way through the pantry. Prednisone causes an increase in appetite, energy and a sense of well-being.

The increase in her pain medicine seems be doing a much better job of keeping Mom comfortable. The spacey feelings will quickly subside. Her Gandhi approach to unwelcome questions will probably reappear from time to time.

Mom and I watched some TV, then it was time to be tucked in and say our prayers. Mom had a good night last night. She did not honk for me, so I have to trust that she was steady enough to go to the bathroom by herself.

Thank you God, for this day so sweet, a pain-free day and a social worker named Marianne. Love, Sue

SEPTEMBER 24, 2001

Yesterday was a good day for Mom. She had her second pain-free day. We enjoyed reading the Sunday paper together. Bryant and Jacob stopped by for a quick visit and promised to return later in the evening. Mom's good friend Mildred, who is 97, called from Missouri. Mom and Mildred enjoy their Sunday chats. Uncle William and Aunt MM stopped by after church to see how Mom was doing. After they left, Mom took an afternoon nap. While she was napping, I did some pruning on some of the flowers in the yard. It is just about time to plant asters, coleus and chrysanthemums. I am so looking forward to fall.

I finished up outside and came in to prepare

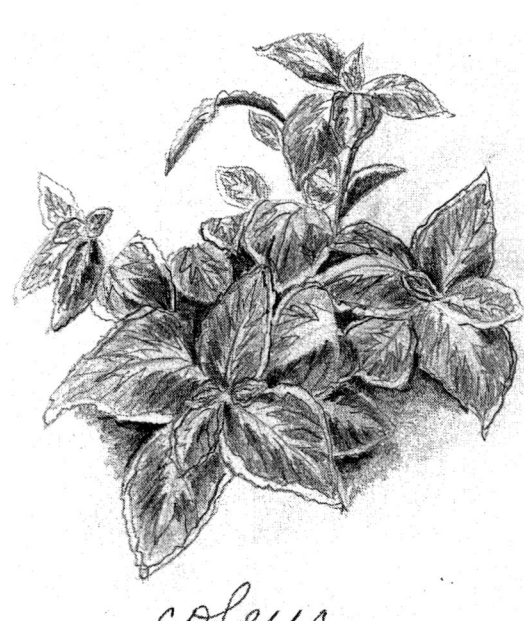

coleus

our Sunday dinner of smothered pork chops, mashed potatoes and carrots. I am always trying to find foods that Mom will find appealing. We watched some TV, then it was time for our evening prayers. Mom had a four-honk night, in laymen's terms, a restless night. Mom was not hurting, but her laxatives kept threatening to kick in. Twice Gracie had to wake me up and tell me she needed a bathroom break. She does not need a horn because she yodels. The cats were surprisingly cooperative. They did not wake me up to go outside, but they were good to go every time I got up. You know, Mom said there would be nights like this.

At six, I was fixing Mom some salt risen toast (thank you, Carol) when Grace wanted to check the backyard. I looked at our thermometer and it read 58°. Well, I flung that door open and discovered it really was 58°. I got so excited and frisky that Grace had to talk me down. She reminded me of our agreement not to do anything that our bodies would make us sorry for. I did run to tell Mom the wonderful news. She did not look happy when I opened the bathroom door and interrupted her concentration with my good news. I know she really is happy that I am happy.

Thank you God, for this day so sweet, Sunday phone calls from old friends and for a 58° morning that tells me fall is on its way. Love, Sue

SEPTEMBER 26, 2001

Mom had a pretty good day yesterday. It was rather low key. We did not have the visitors that we had yesterday. Mom talked on the phone to Becky and Linc. A few times she complained of not feeling well, but could not describe a particular symptom. I am wondering if it is not the prednisone. It can give you a slight sense of agitation. I will have to watch closely for that so the dosage could be adjusted. I have also been observing unusual swelling that will appear in unusual areas. For instance maybe one of Mom's feet will be swollen one time, another time her right hand was swollen, but not her right arm, and now her right cheek is swollen. She looks like she has mumps on one side of her face. She is also having trouble with urination, starting and emptying her bladder. Mom has a stent in her left ureter because the mass had caused it to collapse. It has to be changed every six months. My sister, Becky, said that the last time they did a scan and placed a stent in her left ureter they went on and placed a stent in her right ureter. She recalls Mom's urologist discussing Mom's options. He said that she could do nothing, which would result in kidney failure and a painless death, or they could be aggressive and stent the ureter. Mom chose the stent at that time. I spoke to Christy about Mom's symptoms and asked her if the swelling and urinary symptoms could be related to the impending kidney failure. She said it was possible. She was not sure. She was going to discuss this with the doctor. She did tell Mom that it was her choice to have the stents replaced. It was a simple matter of discharging and readmitting Mom for the one day of her procedure. Mom cannot remain in hospice and have any aggressive treatment. Initially Mom said it did not matter and she would do whatever her children wanted her to do. I told Mom it had to be her decision. She then said let's wait a while. Christy called and said she talked to the doctor and he suggested waiting for now and seeing how it goes. I plan on speaking to her urologist and getting some feedback from him. I will keep you posted as I get more information.

After lunch, Mom took a nap and I went outside and did some pruning and watering. I was in touch with how sad I felt that Mom was not out here with me. I got to thinking how frail and at times unsteady Mom is when she is walking from her bed to the bathroom. At this point, she is not fighting to get out of bed. She has not been in her garden for several days now. All of this is hard. It seems more painful today to watch her withdrawal. I am thankful that she is not hurting.

It really is not all gloom and doom.

Max, our little Pie faced kitty, spent the day sleeping on the pillow next to Mom. I had prepared a meatloaf for dinner which Mom thought was very tasty. We said our prayers and turned in early.

Mom was up twice last night. Thankfully Grace did not have to respond to any calls from nature. I did notice when I was up, that the cats were ready for anything. Ringo had opened up all the lower cabinet doors and was seriously looking for a party. I did not have a party in me at that time.

Thank you God, for this day so sweet, for the comfort and love I feel when I work in my mother's garden, for the blessed assurance I have that your love totally encompasses my mother. Love, Sue

SEPTEMBER 27, 2001

Yesterday was an up-and-down day for Mom. It was a slow start for her, but I got so excited when the outdoor thermometer registered 48°. Grace was able to keep herself balanced, but I was doing the 48° dance of joy. Mom slept through it or at least she pretended to.

Bryant stopped by for a visit. While Bryant was here, Christi came by to check on Mom. It is difficult for me to hear her tell Mom that she does not have to take any medicine other than her pain medicine and her laxatives. I question if they are giving up too soon or I am hanging on too long. I plan on talking to Mom today about whether she wants to let go of any other treatments other than pain. I have the impression that she had things that she still wanted to accomplish. She said last month that she had some unfinished business. If that has changed, I would like to know so that I can be supportive. I am surely not saying that it would be easy, but I would do it.

Marilyn and Judy, Mom's friends, stopped by for an unexpected visit, bearing wonderful muffins and beautiful flowers. Mom really enjoyed their visit.

Lisa, our next-door neighbor, called to say she had a pot of stew for our dinner. Mom had just been talking about how good some stew would be. Mom had a rough time after Marilyn and Judy left. She became nauseated and experienced an increase in pain. This was the first time in a while that her pain was not in control. Things were back in control within an hour. She was even hungry for the stew and cleaned her plate. Just maybe, the prednisone is kicking in.

Mom fell asleep early, so I read Psalm 121. The words spoke to me. "He will never let me stumble, slip or fall. For he is watching, never sleeping."

It was a 4-honk night. Grace even coordinated her visits to the backyard. Every time I got up, the cats were in the kitchen looking wide-eyed and innocent. I know that Ringo is a real prankster. I fully expected to return to bed and find that he had short-sheeted my bed.

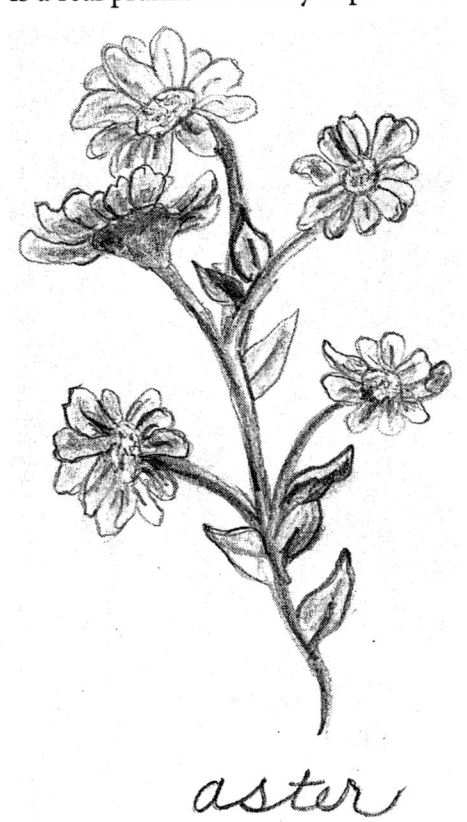

Thank you for this day so sweet, surprise visits from old friends, 48° mornings and the enduring comfort of the Psalms. Love, Sue

SEPTEMBER 29, 2001

Yesterday was a good day for Mom. After our plan of attack on Mom's dreaded constipation problem was a success, we talked about making soapsuds a morning habit. She asked me if I was sure I was up to the task. My mother knows me and my peculiarities and still loves me.

aster

After we were through with our chores, we were walking back to her bed. She asked me how I was doing. I told her I was in good shape as I did not have to institute my emergency evacuation plan. She chuckled and said, "Sue, I love you, but I sometimes wonder about how you see the world." My heart swelled with love for my mother. We have been so blessed to have a mother that loves us, warts and all. I know that I personally have a few prominent warts, but Mother looks right past them. I have been given all I need to have a full rich life. My parents loved me.

Later, Mom decided that she wanted a fried egg sandwich on toasted bread with mayo and a slice of tomato. I think I did good because she licked her plate clean. Christy came while Mom was finishing her sandwich. While Christy was doing her assessment, Mom announced that she was tired and was going to take a nap. Christy looked at me and I shrugged my shoulders. She went on and did Mom's blood-pressure and listened to her chest and her abdomen. Mom never opened her eyes. I could feel a pop quiz coming on, and I was not prepared. Christy went into the kitchen to write her assessment and I went to check my e-mail; OK, I was hiding. Christy sat down and we initially talked about my request and Mom's request that we have some extra oxycontin in the house in case the lollipop does not do the job. Christy kept coming from different angles that Mom really doesn't need pills with the suckers. I knew that behind the decision was a managed-care decision, a money-saving decision. She underestimated my experience in my professional life with patients trying to manipulate me into giving into something that I felt was wrong or not healthy. I think she finally heard me when we agreed to check with the doctor. The plain fact is that we *are* going to get the medicine from a doctor or we will change to another hospice. She changed the subject to Mom's diagnoses. She was not clear that there really is not an accurate diagnosis. The diagnosis is metastatic pancreatic cancer, but it's just a guess. It is not even behaving like pancreatic cancer, in that there's no liver or pancreas involvement. I told her that a year ago the doctor gave Mom three to six months to live. I also did not think that anyone really knows what Mom is in store for, because we are not dealing with a cancer that is behaving typically. I told her that Mom can be a challenge to deal with when she adopts her passive stance. I am a psychiatric nurse and my mother has had me hollering "uncle." Christy said she could see how that might happen after seeing Mom today.

After she left, Mom was done taking her nap. See, I told you. Mom was having her way with poor Christy. When I walked into the room, she had her arms folded across her chest and she was frowning. I asked her what was going on and she said, "I'm disgusted. I just don't like her. She tried to talk you out of the pain pills for me." I tried to comfort her with my conviction that we are going to get that medicine. I ask her if she disliked her because she was a Yankee. Personally, I have nothing against Yankees. She said she did not know why, but she flat-dab did not like her. I am puzzled as to what to do. I asked her if she wanted me to ask for another nurse and she said "no", a new nurse could be worse. Christy is organized, kind and neat, so what do you complain about? I want Mom to have a nurse that will call her "Sugar", talk about her garden, tell her how smart Grace is, ask questions about the photographs on the wall, will give her a hug whenever she comes for a visit and maybe a hug for me and Grace. Christy's bearings are wrapped a little too tight for that. I feel like my hands are tied. I am temporarily at a loss as what to do, if anything. I know if we ask for another nurse it could turn out that we'll wish we had stuck with what we had in the beginning. I also know that when a patient complains to another team member about you, it gets back to you. There aren't any secrets in the team.

When Mom and I said our prayers I included the issue with Christy. It was a one honk night. Mother is still sleeping as I write this. When

I let the critters out, I noticed and felt that it was 50°. This time I did a little jig on the inside, in celebration. I know the cats, in particular Ringo, appreciated my restraint. I think when I dance it scares him. His new water bowl and Mother's new hot pink house dress scare him. So you can imagine what a spontaneous jig would do to his tender psyche.

Thank you God, for this day so sweet, for fried egg sandwiches, for one honk nights and for a mother's love. Love, Sue

OCTOBER 1, 2001

Yesterday was a fair day for Mom. She slept until 9:30. When she woke up, she wanted soup and toast. She drank half a cup and said she was full. Mom said she had some frightening dreams last night about her life being out of control. After we talked, she decided she was still sleepy. I felt like she was withdrawing, but decided then that I would check things out when she woke up. I was going to give her toes a good going over. I left out another solution Becky had to solve Mom's toes curling problem. It was rat paper—like flypaper but for rats. It is real sticky and we could put the paper on the bottom of Mom's feet and straighten out her toes. We then could cut around her feet leaving a snowshoe effect. Diane cracked up when I told her about Becky's idea. We are talking about our delicate baby sister.

Mom finally woke up about 1:15 p.m. I took a deep breath and told her that I felt like we needed to make sure our lines of communication were open. I was holding us to the promise we made to each other that we did not have to be alone on this journey. We could talk about what scares us and what makes us happy. I needed to talk about some things that I was feeling sad and overwhelmed about. She sat up and said, "Let's talk."

I began with how important it was to keep separate what I wanted and what she wanted. My number one want is that she has exactly what she wants and needs. This is her journey, and I am here walking with her. I told her that I had a big fear that I needed to tell her about. I told her that I was concerned with how stable she was when walking and it had declined sharply in the last few weeks. I was concerned that she was slowly withdrawing and would end up in a fetal position in bed. I was concerned that there was something I was not doing. If she was tired and wanted to do nothing to extend her life, I would honor her wish. What I am struggling with is the quality of the life she has left. She said that she was not ready to give in and how she was walking was of great concern to her. I told her about one more concern I had, her toes curling up. I uncovered her feet and there they were all clinched up in a knot. I asked her if she could straighten her toes. All of a sudden she had all of her toes flared out. She said, "I have told people that I don't know how to relax. You and Diane clinched your toes." I only clinch my toes when I'm wearing sandals. I was relieved nothing permanent had happened. She suggested that I rub her feet and see if I couldn't get them to relax. I performed that rub with great enthusiasm. I asked Mom what she would like for lunch and she said french fried potatoes. She cleaned her plate and decided to take a nap. Later, when she was waking up, Uncle William and Aunt MM came by for a visit. Mom had a birthday gift for her. I got a call from my good friend, Pernell. He is a nurse that I worked with and he also saved my life by getting me to the hospital when I was in acute respiratory failure. He plans on driving in from Louisiana Monday morning, so he could see Mom and say goodbye to us before he shipped off. He is in the reserves and will have to leave Tuesday.

Bryant stopped by for a visit with Mom. He is in the process of packing, in preparing to move to a duplex in Carrollton. While he was here, I mixed up my famous hush puppies, one of Mom's personal favorites, to go with Becky's stew. I took Mom's plate to her and she said, "Sue, I have to go to the bathroom." She was so shaky when I was getting her out of bed. We finally made it to the bathroom. She was clutching the sink. She said she felt numb like she was floating out of her body. I was able to get her back in bed. Mother looked so tense, like she could break into pieces, her eyes were clamped shut and she said that she couldn't talk. I could not, for the life of me, figure out what was going on. She had some of the classic signs of a full-blown panic attack, the numbness, floating outside your body. I decided to put an Atavan under her tongue to see if it would help. She suddenly asked me to call Marilyn to come and sit with her. I told her I could sit with her and was not clear on why she felt like we needed help. She also said, "Sue, please don't leave me." She did not answer. I went on and put up her dinner, but she needed to take her pain medicine and her laxatives. I gave them to her one at a time with shaved ice. She never opened her eyes.

I was standing there looking at Mom when the phone rang. I was so pleased to discover it was my cousin, Margaret. We talked for some time and I ended up crying a lot. I was surprised by my tears. I was not aware that I had been storing them up. She was so comforting to me. She talked about how hard it was to watch her Mother's body shut down. It was something that she could not fix. She suggested that I listen very carefully to what Mom was saying and what her body was saying. Her body might really be at a point where it couldn't be fixed with just one more pill. She suggested that I pray about this and an answer would come. She said all the things that I so needed to hear.

When I went to check on Mom she had relaxed little bit and said she would be okay now and to go on to bed. We said our prayers and I tucked her in for the night. It was a two honk night.

When we got up at six, Mom said she was hungry for my dinner. I asked her if she would rather have ham and eggs. She decided on the stew, even though it was morning. I was standing in the bathroom with Mother, when I asked her about what she thought was going on last night. She looked me square in the eye and said, "I thought I was dying." I shook my head and asked her why on earth she did not tell me that bit of information. She said, "Well, I thought you would figure it out!" I could not control myself, I busted out laughing. I apologized for my outburst, but by this time she was smiling. I told her that when people describe floating sensations, I think they might be having a panic attack. That is why I put an Atavan under her tongue. We had gotten back to bed by this time, and I asked her if she thought it was peculiar for me to be poking pills in her mouth last night, while she thought she was dying. We both had a chuckle. I made her promise me if she ever feels like she's dying again, because I don't like to have to guess what is going on, she might give me a clue. I would want to say goodbye. She was afraid her other children might get in an accident trying to get there as fast as they could. We finished our chat and she finished her stew and Hush Puppies. So I came in here to write this long letter.

Thank you God, for this day so sweet, for heart-to-heart talks with my mother, my hush puppies recipe, for a just in the nick of time call from my cousin Margaret, and for shared laughter with my mom. Love, Sue

Hush Puppies

1 cup corn meal
1 tsp garlic salt
1/4 tsp soda
dash pepper
1 small onion finely chopped
1 stalk celery
½ cup buttermilk
    Stir together
    Cook in hot oil

OCTOBER 2, 2001

Mom had a great day yesterday after our talk about not making me guess whether she was dying or not. She decided to sit in her recliner for while. It seemed like a light had been turned on inside Mother. She asked for two recipe books that hold many handwritten recipes from herself, her mother, family, friends and magazines. She was looking for a recipe for a 30-day cake. She and Carol had talked about this earlier and she was determined to find it.

While Mom was sitting up, Marilyn called to say she had read my note and wanted to cook something and bring it over. I told her that Mom loved her vegetable soup. She said she would be by later with soup from her kitchen. My friend, Pernell, called to say it would be later this afternoon before he could get to Dallas, but he was coming. I am so touched. He had worked all last night and would have to turn around and leave at 4 in the morning so he could work his evening shift. He doesn't know when he will be shipped off and wanted to be sure that he had a chance to say goodbye to Mom. He is like having another brother.

Mom was hungry and polished off a sizable number of chips with her favorite salsa. So far, she has had stew, hush puppies and chips and salsa before lunch. Before I knew it, Marilyn was here with a big container of her vegetable soup and flowers from her garden. She had included some aromatic basil and oregano. Mom and I both rubbed the leaves and smelled our fingers and were immediately filled with the love that Marilyn has for her garden and for how thoughtful she was to add such wonderfully satisfying fragrances from her garden. She sat with Mom and they talked about Mom's experience last night. Marilyn told me that if Mom wanted me to call her to come over I was to do exactly that. It did not matter if I understood why Mom was making that request. I immediately felt so comforted by her words. I have written about how wonderful it is to have such good friends and this is the perfect illustration of what friends do for each other.

They were talking about recipes when Christy came by for her visit. Mom did not take a nap during her assessment. Marilyn went and walked in Mother's garden, while Christy was here. In fact, she fed the birds while she was out there. Mom was very direct with Christy about wanting the ability to choose whether she uses a sucker or pill to control her breakthrough pain. In fact, she told her that she was eager to get the assessment completed so she could continue her visit with Marilyn.

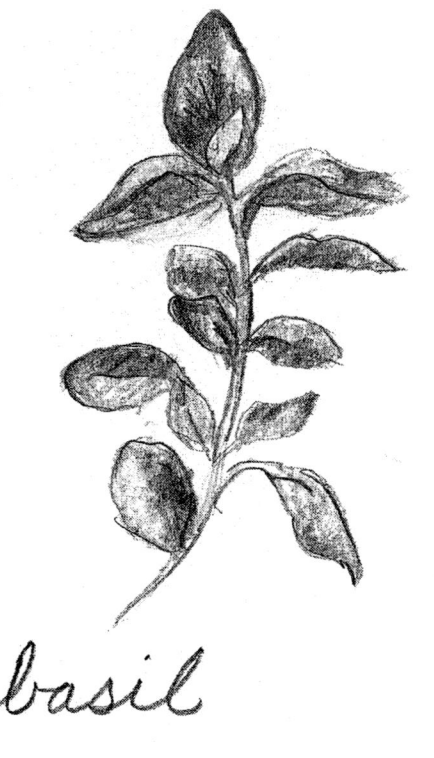

basil

Pat, our neighbor across the street, came over to get a list of a few things I needed for Pernell's visit. She said a quick hello to Mom then left to go to work. Mom was beginning to tire, so Marilyn said goodbye. Before she left, she came into my room and we talked for while. She offered to stay with Mom so Lynda, Pat and I can go to the State fair. I have been wanting to go for years, and it had never worked out. When Marilyn got home, she e-mailed me about assisting Mom in completing her written personal history. She also suggested a taped conversation with Mom talking about her memories. I responded with an enthusiastic "yes!" I know that it would lift Mom's spirits.

I got a call from Lisa telling me that she had homemade chicken noodle soup for our dinner. Mom slept until Carolyn came to help her with her bath. By the time Mom got in bed, she was asleep when her head hit the pillow. I woke her at 7 p.m. to eat some soup. While we were eating, Pernell finally arrived. It was so good to see him. He also got a bowl of soup, and we began to catch up with each other's lives. It was soon time for Mom to go to sleep so we gathered around the bed and said our prayers together. Pernell kissed Mom goodnight and we went into the other room to talk. Pernell is an assistant chaplain with the reserves. He is prepared to go wherever he is needed. He promised to send us his mailing address when he gets to where they are sending him. It was soon time for us to turn in, since he was having to get up so early to leave.

Mom had a 1-honk night. I got up at 4 a.m. to wake Pernell and also be sure that I had a chance to say goodbye to him. It seems fitting he was here in time for evening prayers.

Thank you God, for this day so sweet, for the loving support of a friend named Marilyn, for our neighbors, for the chance to have Pernell share our evening prayers, and for the feeling that we are surrounded by your angels. Love, Sue

OCTOBER 3, 2001

Yesterday was a good day for Mom. She slept till 10 a.m. Uncle William, Aunt MM and Lee stopped by to drop off our dinners she had cooked for us. Janet, the hospice chaplain, came by to visit with Mom. At the beginning, Mom and I talked with Janet about Mom not feeling comfortable with Christy's style. I also brought up the apparent control struggle that has developed with the medical director and myself about Mom's PRN (this stands for "as needed") pain medicine. I want her to have the opportunity to choose between the pills or the suckers. When he renewed Mom's medicine, she received a whole bunch of oxycontin and only four suckers. Mom uses between one and two suckers a day. I know that it is a money thing, but it is not my problem whether they make a profit on Mom's care. I firmly believe that Mom should be able to choose between the two different methods of break-through pain control. I told Janet that if this was not resolved to our satisfaction, I would go to another hospice. She felt sure that it all can be worked out. I am to talk to Marianne today about having another nurse besides Christy for Mom. If I develop a reputation, so be it. Mom is going to have the best care available. I will do what Becky does and start asking for the spelling of their middle name. For some reason that question usually results in a dramatic increase in the quality of customer service provided. I know when Becky asked me to spell my middle name, I moved from the position where I was only capable of passing water to being able to walk on water. If you don't ask for what you need and want, you can be sure not to get anything. So I remind myself that I have to be clear about my expectations. Becky is truly a good role model for that behavior.

After Janet left, Mom sat up in the recliner and had some vegetable soup. She surprised me by asking if I was up to a walk in her garden. We managed that without a problem. She had an opportunity to see how beautiful her sedum and mums looked blooming together. After she came in, she decided to take a short nap. Before she laid down for a nap, Lynda called from the lake to make sure Mom was doing ok. The short nap turned into a long one, and I woke Mom so she could eat her dinner. After dinner, she enjoyed reading her mail. We said our prayers early and she fell asleep shortly after I kissed her goodnight. It was a 2-honk night. Grace was thoughtful to coordinate her toileting needs with Mom's.

Thank you God, for this day so sweet, for homemade vegetable soup, for the gift of confidence in working with the complex system to get the best care possible for Mom, for the blessing of having a baby sister named Becky who continues to teach me something new every day, and for a walk in the garden with my mother. Love, Sue

OCTOBER 5, 2001

Yesterday was a fairly quiet day for Mom, but a busy day for the house. Cil and Delbert came over. Delbert came to begin work on the brick wall around the patio. Cil and I played seven games of Skip Bo and I won all seven games. I have never won more than two games at any one time. It was really a fun time. Cil and I talk every day. She has emphysema and is also on continuous oxygen. We met in rehab and became fast friends.

Mom did not feel like she could sit up and play cards with us. I think she was enjoying the downtime from all the questions. After Cil and Delbert left, I went to check on Mom and she was awake. She asked me if I wasn't scared of Cil. I was shocked. I asked her to explain what she was talking about. She related that she had heard Cil talk loudly about how she hated Highland Park teachers and how she kept hollering "hot and cold." I told Mom I was sure she had been dreaming this and I was not scared of Cil.

She decided to get up and check out the progress on the patio. Afterwards, she got cleaned up and sat in her recliner and looked at catalogs. I made a mental note to decrease her prednisone. I am sure that it is feeding into the bizarre dreams in the undercurrent of her agitation. I had great hopes that the prednisone was going to have a more positive impact than it has. She ate a bowl full of salsa and chips. The prednisone has certainly helped her appetite.

Mom and I ate dinner and watched TV together. Mom was surprised when Diane called and chatted. I overheard her tell Diane that she was hearing and seeing things that weren't there. I asked her to tell me what she was hearing and seeing. She replied "the usual stuff." I am really, really cutting back on the prednisone. It was soon time for bed and we said our prayers and she was tucked in tight for the night.

Around 11:30 Mom honked and when I got to her room I discovered a bowl of salsa and a bag of chips. She said she didn't remember getting up and getting them. She looked distressed and told me that she was having bad dreams. She expressed fear that she was destitute and alone. I comforted her and reminded her that she was safe and secure. I also gave her an Ambien to help her go back to sleep. I tucked her in extra tight.

I was awake at 5, watching a movie when Mom honked and I went to check on her. She was sitting on the edge of the bed and I asked her if she was ready to go to the bathroom. She said that she needed help in getting her covers smoothed out because she just returned from the bathroom. My heart leapt into my throat again, because she is so unsteady when she walks. I asked her why she didn't honk for me. She told me that she found herself in the bathroom and had no memory of how she got there. There is a horn in the bathroom that she could have used to alert me. I am truly amazed she has not fallen. I am hoping that later we can talk and get some of this sorted out.

Thank you God, for this day so sweet, for an angel named Delbert, for Christmas catalogs, for keeping my mother safe through the night and for giving me the words to comfort my mother. Love, Sue

OCTOBER 6, 2001

Yesterday was a better day for Mom. She started off with asking me for an Ativan because she was hungry. I asked her if she was anxious. She said no, she was hungry for breakfast. She ended up eating half of her breakfast. After breakfast, Delbert came over to work on the brick wall. I am so overwhelmed by his generosity. Mom was in good spirits and seemed to enjoy her morning shows. It got real overcast outside which made her room darker. I think that triggered an unplanned nap. Lynda surprised me by stopping by. She had just driven in from the lake and was wanting to check on Mom. We visited and I finally decided to wake Mom at 2 p.m. so she would not feel like she had slept the day away.

She was very happy to see Lynda. When asked what she would like for lunch, Mom smiled real big and said a Schlotsky's. Lynda turned right around and went and got a Schlotsky's sandwich. Mom said she felt better at that moment than she had in felt a long time. She sat in the kitchen and ate half the sandwich. While she was eating, she decided that she wanted to cook stew. We needed stew meat, so Lynda turned around and went to the store to pick up the necessary ingredients. Mom prepared the carrots and gave the rest of the directions to Lynda when she returned from the store.

Caroline had arrived to help her with her bath. So the stew preparation was interrupted. Lynda asked me if I was okay. I was aware of feeling a mixture of sad and happy feelings, watching Mom in the kitchen. I was happy to see her once again in the kitchen. I was also sad at the reminder of how empty the kitchen has felt since she has been in bed. There is so much that I don't know when it comes to Mom's secret ways of cooking certain dishes. I love the way she does her coleslaw. I have seen her make it hundreds of times, but never paid attention to details. I made a stab at making her blender slaw. But I was not successful. Maybe today Mom can show me how she makes it perfect every time.

She took a short nap after all the activity in the kitchen and getting her bath. I woke her so she could have her dinner. We watched TV before turning in. I tucked her in tight and we said our prayers.

It was a 1-honk night. When I went to let Grace out I was met with 47° weather. For some reason, Grace left quickly to check her yard, as I commenced my 47° dance of joy. The cats looked at each other and asked if this was going to be a part of every fall and winter morning. I smiled and said, "Probably! Just wait and see what happens when there is snow and ice!" They are not the only ones that can feel frisky. I was so in the mood, that while I sit here and type this note, I am listening to Christmas music. It seemed very appropriate to me.

Thank you God for this day so sweet, for Mom waking up hungry, for my friend Lynda's visit, for Schlotsky's sandwiches, for Mom's return to her kitchen and for Christmas music. Love, Sue

OCTOBER 7, 2001

Yesterday was a good day for Mom. Delbert came by to continue to work on the brick wall. Mom slept till 9, then Uncle William and Aunt MM stopped by for a short visit. As they were leaving, Carol arrived with hugs, wonderful stories, a wonderful wooden bear for Mom and a whole bunch of Christmas catalogs. We enjoyed hearing about her adventures at the State Fair. After Carol left, Mom decided to take a short nap before Becky and Tom came for their Saturday visit. I took some time and looked at some of the catalogs. I had a near Christmas experience while I looked at Carol's catalogs.

Becky, Tom and Sherri arrived with groceries and a sour cream pound cake. Tom started some repair work on the kitchen chairs and Becky and I sorted through the groceries. I was in talking with Mom, when Lynda snuck in and surprised me. She came over to see what was going on with Mom and if there was anything she could do. I started getting ready to go out and Becky started her cleaning. The car battery was dead, so Lynda let me borrow her car, so I did not have to wait for AAA. I really enjoyed my time out. I picked up some fall color for Mom's room, while I was out shopping.

When I returned, I found Mom sitting up in bed going through her pajama drawer. She was sorting out what was too big for her to wear now. Becky had done Mom's hair, Tom had put the air-conditioner in the kitchen window, Sherri had made a banner for Mom's room and Lynda had added the finishing touches to the stew. It felt good to come home.

Mom was talking about needing to make some changes. She was not clear as to what changes she was talking about. I guess when she's ready to tell me she will let me know. She enjoyed reading her e-mails from Diane, Jenny and Marilyn. The mail also brought notes from Aunt FiFi.

Mom and I were both tired, so we turned in early after we said our prayers. She did not honk for me last night. I found evidence of her being up, the walker was moved and her cane was hanging on her bedside table. When I let Grace out, the thermostat read 43°. I came back in and put on Christmas music and typed out my morning note.

Thank you God, for this day so sweet, for Carol and her gift of Christmas catalogs, for a day to play, for keeping Mom safe last night, and for the comfort that a visit from family and friends brings to one's heart. Love, Sue

Sour Cream Pound Cake

2 sticks butter
3 cups sugar
6 eggs separated
1/4 tsp soda
1 cup sour cream
3 cups sifted flour
1 tsp almond extract
1 tsp vanilla
    Cream butter and sugar
    Add egg yolks one at a time and beat well
    Add flour and sour cream alternately and blend well
    Add extract and fold in stiffly beaten egg whites
    Pour in greased and floured tube pan
    Bake at 300° for 1½ hours

OCTOBER 8, 2001

Yesterday was a good day for Mom. She slept till 10 a.m. There was evidence that she had been up during the night. I have to trust that she feels steady enough to use her walker by herself. She does appear to be steadier when she walks and is not so anxious that I hold her tightly as she walks.

I knew this was going to be a good day when I found the Mafia movie on cable. I have this attraction to this type of movie, but I rarely watch all of the movie, because of the violence. I have developed a "third eyelid" that protects me from any of the bloodshed. I think I am so attracted to Mafia movies because they dramatize the strength of family and loyalty to family. I know it is twisted loyalty, because one never really knows when you are going for that long car ride. It is a modern-day fairy tale. Not many people knew of my weakness for gangster movies until now. When I am feeling stressed the first thing that brings me comfort is some Jesus music and prayer. Mafia movies and gardening shows like the *Victory Garden* also have a different kind of calming effect. I remember when Mom was so sick five years ago, I watched a gardening show on dirt. I had to use my third eyelid because of the worms. All to say, the hour spent learning about dirt was calming…go figure. I still don't understand that.

Anyway, Delbert brought Cil with him when he came to work on the patio wall. We were getting ready to play Skip-Bo when Mom decided to join us in a game. I was so excited I could hardly contain myself. After playing a game, Mom sat at the table and ate her lunch while Cil and I played another game of Skip-Bo. She decided after the second game to return to bed and take a nap. She was having trouble with being sleepy.

I had to wake Mom so she could eat her dinner. She also had some e-mails to read. We were both hungry for chili dogs, so we had chili dogs. While we were waiting for dinner to get hot, Mom wanted me to call Gary and Sue next door. She wanted Gary to come check out our heater and she was concerned that she had not seen Sue in a while. Mom and Sue have had a close and loving relationship since Mom and Dad moved into this house. Mom had told me that she was sure that Sue was probably having a hard time with the idea that she was in hospice. Sue lost her mother about a year ago, and last month, her favorite sister-in-law died. When I talked with her about Mom, she admitted that she was having a big struggle with the idea of losing someone else that she loves. She told me that she was going to get a grip and come see Mom. I told her anytime she wanted to come would be fine with Mom. Mom was pleased that Sue had talked about her fears.

After dinner we watched a little TV and decided to turn in. We said our prayers and I kissed her goodnight. She didn't honk for me last night. She is still asleep as I write this note.

Thank you God, for this day so sweet, for the game of Skip-Bo with Mom, for the beautiful weather, for friends and neighbors like Sue and for our world that contains many odd and wonderful things that offer comfort. Love, Sue

OCTOBER 9, 2001

Sorry about sending four letters, but my computer seemed to have developed a stutter. Yesterday was a pretty good day for Mom. She slept in, which seems to be becoming a pattern. Delbert arrived early to finish the patio wall. After Mom had her toast, she dozed off again. Lynda arrived around 11. She was going to run some errands for Mom and me. She noticed that Mom was watching a different soap from her favorite. Mom did not seem to notice the difference. When Lynda told me this, my eyes filled up with tears. This is really so hard. Her eyes look so weary. I was concerned that Mom was trying to cover up some confusion so I decided to approach her. I first had to get my tears under control. I know Diane, it is okay for Mom to see my tears and she does, but I did not want to overwhelm her when I talked with her.

After Lynda left to run errands, I sat down at the end of the bed and asked her if she was having trouble organizing her thoughts. I told her that if she was, I did not want her to hide it from me because it would be difficult for me to tolerate the idea that she was scared and confused. She said she wasn't sure if it was Monday or Tuesday. Mom talked about how it worried her not to be able to keep track of the days of the week. She decided to get out of bed and go outside and check out the patio wall. We sat out there for about thirty minutes and listened to the birds and the water from the fountain. After we came back and she sat down at the table to catch her breath, I ask Mom if she felt sad. She said yes, and she didn't know why. She asked me if she could have an Ativan. After I gave her the medication she told me that it was ok to cry. I told her that I felt so sad that I did not know how to make things better. She told me that there were things that were beyond my control. I really needed that reminder. It is so good to clear the air. Mom and I talked about keeping true to our pledge to talk about our concerns that either of us have. I hugged her and she got up and walked to her room to sit in her recliner for a while.

Lynda returned with tacos for lunch. Mom wanted to finish cleaning out her pajama drawer. After Lynda left, Kathy, the new nurse arrived to check on Mom. I liked her immediately. She wanted to know all about Grace Elizabeth. Mom seemed to warm up to her and talked about her children. Kathy didn't call Mom "Sugar", but she came pretty durn close. I am so relieved. She will be back on Thursday. Mom was soon asleep after Kathy left.

Delbert finished the wall around the patio and it looks beautiful. Mom will be so pleased when she sees it. I woke her for dinner and we sat at the kitchen table. We watched the Antique Road Show together, and it was soon time to say our prayers and turn in for the night.

Thank you God, for this day so sweet, for Delbert who added to the beauty of Mom's garden, for sending a nurse named Kathy and for eating dinners at the kitchen table with Mom. Love, Sue

OCTOBER 10, 2001

Yesterday was a sleepy day for Mom. I awoke her at 9 a.m. so she could take her scheduled pain medicine. She was hungry so I fixed her a poached egg and bacon. I was pleased when she ate all of it. She was having some breakthrough pain, so I gave her the PRN oxycontin. I knew it would make her sleepy, but it is important that she not hurt. I sat and watched her sleep for a long time. I am already feeling lonely.

As I thumbed through the Sunday coupons, I was painfully reminded of how long it has been since she has been to the grocery store. There is a Southern Living magazine on her bedside table that she has yet to look at. I spent some time putting some garlands of fall leaves around her mirror to give her room the seasonal look, and maybe bring a smile to her lips. Last Saturday Sherri put up some Halloween lights. Mom and I are both pack rats and Becky really is good-natured about straightening up Mom's nest. Becky will have to have major medication when she sees what I have planned for Christmas.

Mom's kitties, Ringo and Max, take turns sleeping in shifts on Mom's bed. Maybe there is something about that bed which puts you to sleep. I finally woke Mom at 1 p.m. so she could eat some lunch. She ate all of her hot roast beef sandwich and decided to get cleaned up. When she returned bed, she looked at her e-mails from Diane and Jenny. She also read the note that her sister FiFi sends every day. I told her that I had prepared corn pudding for dinner using her recipe.

The show *Crossing Over* was on TV. It is a show about a psychic that reportedly can talk to people that have died. I asked Mom if she believed that he was really talking to people that have crossed over. I also asked her if she thought her mother had ever tried to communicate with her. She responded with a simple "no" to both questions. I talked to Becky about her response and she was surprised because she has vivid memories of Mom feeling like Grandmother was standing at the foot of her bed. It makes me wonder if she has forgotten those memories or she is just not wanting to talk about it. She was rather quiet and didn't seem to want to chat. It wasn't long before she was asleep again.

Bryant called and I knew that Mom had wanted to talk to him, so I woke her up. He has been busy moving and it had been awhile since they had talked. She was asleep shortly after she finished talking with Bryant.

The mail came and my Willie Nelson *Amazing Grace* CD had finally arrived! I put it on and listened to him singing *Farther Along*. I feel so comforted by the words. It was one of the songs they sang at Daddy's funeral. I resisted the temptation to wake up Mom. I was feeling so lonesome for her. I became aware of how I was really missing the sounds and the smells that would accompany dinnertime when Mom was in the kitchen. There were good smells coming from the kitchen, but it was not the same. I decided to wake her because it would soon be time for dinner. Mom surprised me and cleaned her plate at dinner. She was still not feeling like chatting, so we watched some TV. I tucked her and we said our prayers. She did not honk for me last night.

Thank you God, for this day so sweet, for Mom's appetite, for having a hand written recipe for Mom's corn pudding, for a reassuring call from Bryant, for garlands of fall color that remind us of nature's beauty and which reminds my sister Becky of what is in store for her in December. Love, Sue

OCTOBER 11, 2001

Yesterday was another sleepy day for Mom. Mom woke up around 8:30. Her tummy was bothering her. After she took some medicine, she was ready for breakfast. She asked for an egg in a hole and bacon. I was pleased when she cleaned her plate. I told her that Janet, the chaplain was coming for a visit. She smiled and said she was going to get a quick nap. I caught myself wondering if this is how it is going to be…me waking her up to go to the bathroom and to eat and drink some water and her falling back to sleep.

Janet and Kathy, her new nurse, arrived at the same time. They really liked the garlands and the pumpkin lights. It sure felt good when they both commented on how obvious it was that Mom was loved when they saw all the cards and special touches in her room. Mom put on her Halloween costume for them. We all had a big chuckle. Her Halloween costume consists of these purple glasses, with bushy pink eyebrows attached to the rims and an awfully big, green, bumpy witch's nose, with snaggleteeth. They spent quite a bit of time with Mom, but she dozed through most of the visit. My eyes filled with tears when Kathy asked me how many hours Mom was awake during the day. I told her maybe four hours. I shocked myself, when I heard myself say four hours. I knew she was sleeping a lot, but I had not really absorbed the amount of time she was sleeping. Kathy hugged me and said she would see Mom on Monday. Janet also left after she said a prayer with Mom.

Uncle William and Aunt MM stopped by for a short visit. Mom had trouble waking up enough to see them. Lynda arrived with some groceries as they were leaving. She and I visited while Mom slept. I, again, became tearful about what was happening to Mom. I am not holding back today because there is no reason not to cry. As we would say in psychiatric terms, my mood was congruent to my effect. It is all part of the grief process.

I woke Mom around 1:30, so she could go to the bathroom and eat. Lynda helped her to the bathroom, while I was heating up her lunch. She did not seem to have much of an appetite today. She was asleep shortly after she finished her lunch. I decided to lay down for a few minutes and Lynda left to run some errands. I got up and did a few chores around the house, then I started getting dinner together. I decided to wake up Mom at 5:30, so she could at least get a full glass of water down. She was fairly cooperative, but seemed to doubt my estimate of how much she is drinking. We went on and had dinner, which she ate only a small portion of, but she did get a full glass of water down. I told her how much I had been missing her. She responded by telling me how much she had been missing me. After she finished eating, it was no time before she was asleep again. I did wake her, so we could say our prayers together. She slept all night.

Thank you God, for this day so sweet, for Kathy's hug, for shared tears, for those wonderful purple glasses and for your promise to bring comfort to those who are grieving. Love, Sue

Egg in a Hole

eggs
bread
butter

    Melt butter in a small skillet
    Use a juice glass to cut a hole in the center of a slice of bread
    Keep the circle that is removed
    Place bread in the skillet
    Break the egg in the hole
    Cook till partially done, then turn and cook to your liking
    You can also cook the cupped-out bread

OCTOBER 12, 2001

Mom was a little more awake yesterday. She woke around 9 a.m. She thought French toast would taste good, so I prepared some for her. She ate about half of her breakfast. She was able to stay awake and watched some morning TV. I was supposed to go to the fair Thursday, but it was too rainy for my lungs. Thankfully, Mom was more cooperative in drinking a glass of water with her breakfast. Lynda stopped by with some salt risen bread. Mom decided it would be fun if we all played a game of Skip-Bo. Mom won the game. It was a fairly long game and Mom was tired after the first game and decided to lay down. She was asleep in no time. Lynda and I played another game, which she won. We both decided that we needed to get some chores done, so she left to run her errands and I folded laundry.

Mom slept till 5 and I woke her up, so she could go to the bathroom and drink some water. While dinner was heating, I tried to engage her in conversation. She seemed so detached. I tried not to ask yes/no questions, but that was usually the response to my questions. I know that detachment is one of the stages of dying. I guess people go through stages at their own pace. Mom does seem to still be able to track the activity around the house. Her eyes at times have a vacant forty-yard stare. I told her again how lonesome I have been for her and she said the same. She wished she could stay awake. I wonder sometimes if she isn't just retreating into sleep. I keep coming back to my fear, that she is choosing to sleep to escape from something. I have tried to figure out what she might be retreating from. It could be that she is choosing not to fight the sedative effects of her pain medicine. I worry that this marathon sleeping is impacting her kidneys. She only urinated four times yesterday and it appeared concentrated. At this point, I don't think that her urologist would consider putting a stent in her ureter which would keep her kidney from dying. Her urologist told her six months ago that if she opted not to go with a stent placement, renal failure was a fairly painless way to die. I would like to have some blood work done, but I am told that this is probably not an option. I might insist. I would like to know what her BUN and creatinine is (they tell you how your kidneys are functioning).

Anyway, after dinner, Bryant, Jacob and Sara came for a visit. Mom was happy they had been able to come by because it had been about two weeks since she had seen them. They had been so involved in moving to Carrollton and getting established in their new schools. Mom and I watched some of *Who Wants to be a Millionaire* and then it was time for our prayers.

She slept through the night. I am excited because I am going to the fair this morning with Lynda and Kelley. I have not been to the fair since I was in college. Marilyn is coming to stay with Mom while I am gone. I am sure that I will have lots of stories when I return home.

Thank you God, for this day so sweet, for a game of Skip-Bo with Mom and Lynda, for Marilyn who is staying with Mom while I go to the fair with Lynda and Kelley, for Bryant, Jacob and Sara's visit and for blessing me with sisters who can tell by my voice that I am feeling sad or stressed and know the words to lift me up. Love, Sue

OCTOBER 13, 2001

Yesterday Mom and I both had a wonderful day. Marilyn came over and stayed with Mom and I went to the fair with Lynda and Kelley. Marilyn and Mom had planned to work on her memory book, recipes and Marilyn was going to tape Mom as she talked about her memories. I did have a little trouble separating from Mom. I knew she was in good hands with Marilyn. I left a phone number where I could be reached and kissed Mom goodbye.

What a day we had at the fair. There were funnel cakes, Fletcher's corny dogs, fried green tomatoes and corn on the cob. There were a lot of other things we did besides eat. The weather was beautiful. We saw every kind of goat imaginable. Then there was the dog show with the dogs showing off what they did best. We saw all of the different jams, pickles, pictures, quilts and crafts that had won ribbons. We saw a painted wooden display of two cows standing and they had holes, where you stick your head through and get your picture made. I was able to persuade Lynda and Kelley to pose. Kelley got in a wheelchair race with an older lady and her husband. We won and no one was hurt. She and Lynda both had a way with pushing the wheel chair. At times we would twirl, jiggle or zoom along. They were good sports about pushing my chariot around. I did not start off in the wheelchair, but I soon got tired and that required more oxygen, so the wheelchair helped me to last as long as Lynda and Kelley could last. Lynda was dealing with a painful blister on her little toe. The Bonnie and Clyde exhibit was fascinating. We found out that Sparkman Hillcrest Funeral Home buried Clyde Barrow because they were handing out funeral fans. Of course, we all had to have a fan. I have a thing about fans, so I was real happy.

We went and saw all the different booths that were selling products that would change your life forever, by straightening out your arches, by making housework a pleasure and potions that would detoxify your system. I bought some pear jam and green tomato pickles for Mom. I knew that would put a smile on her lips. We then walked across the grounds to get to the miniature White House exhibit. On our way to the exhibit, we were treated to a parade of the Marine Marching Band. Everyone clapped and yelled, as they passed by. We then got in a long line to see the exhibit. It was truly amazing. They had china and momentos from each President. We then got to see the magnificent miniature White House. This will probably be the closest I will ever get to having an idea of what that amazing house is like. They had several TV sets that were showing current news coverage. The phones rang and there were fires in the fireplaces. They even had George and Laura

Bush's pictures on the wall. We did not have time to see all of the other exhibits because it was getting late, but we did see FDR's limo. It was olive green and had a ramp for his wheelchair and there was a space in the limo for his wheelchair to sit next to the back-seat. On our way to the car we stopped at a first aid station and got Lynda a band aid for her little toe. We also made a final stop to get Mom a chili cheese dog and Kelley a caramel apple. As we were driving out of the parking lot, it had started raining. We had timed it just right. When we got home, Bryant and the kids were there. Marilyn had had to leave, so Bryant said he could stay till I got home. Mom ate her chili dog right away. She said that she had a wonderfully full day with Marilyn. I was surprised when she told me that she had not slept while I was gone. Marilyn called to tell me that she had taped Mom talking about her memories of World War II. They had looked at recipe books and Mom's aide, Carolyn, came to help Mom, and the social worker, Marianne, came by for a visit. I was so happy that Mom and Marilyn enjoyed the day together. I am sure that I will never forget how wonderful this day had been for Mom and me. I really, really needed a day like this to recharge my batteries.

Mom and I said our prayers and I tucked her in for the night. She appears to have slept through the night.

Thank you God, for this day so sweet and for the gift of a wondrous Friday and our friends Marilyn, Lynda and Kelley who made it all possible. Love, Sue

OCTOBER 14, 2001

Yesterday was another good day for Mom and me. We both slept in, after our big day yesterday. I was still in my nightgown when Uncle William, Aunt MM and Lee stopped by with strawberries for Mom. She was in the kitchen, taking a peek at her garden when they arrived. She did return to bed shortly after they left. Mom and I both smiled when we talked about Becky, Tom and Sherri coming for their Saturday visit. They arrived with groceries and Schlotsky sandwiches for all. Becky, Sherri and I ate our sandwiches in Mom's room. We all had a wonderful visit. I was full of stories from the fair, Mom was talking about meeting her new hospice volunteer, Fausto, and Becky was being the mischievous little sister. It felt so good to have all of us in that room, laughing and reminiscing. Becky then got into some serious vacuuming and Tom and Sherri went and ran an errand. I had the luxury of puttering around my room. I started looking through Carol's catalogs again for that perfect Christmas present. I have found quite a few things that I would like to order. After Becky finished "freshening" the house, and Tom had hung my Halloween windsock up, and Sherri had hugged her Granny, it was time for them to head home.

Mom told me to bring her a stack of catalogs to look at. I swear I got so excited that if I had a tail to chase, I would have been chasing it. While we were looking at catalogs, I put on some potatoes to cook to go with the roast beef and gravy that Becky had brought. After dinner, we were surprised with a visit from Bryant. We all watched the *Touched by An Angel* show about Andrew, the Angel of Death and his experiences. I did comment on how comforting the show was and Mom agreed. Mom was ready to be tucked in for the night and she had Bryant to come get me, so I could show him our routine. While I was tucking her in, she asked him if he was paying attention. Bryant told Mom that he could tuck her in next time. After we said our prayers, he left for home. Mom appeared to sleep through the night.

Thank you God,, for this day so sweet, for the wonderful Saturday chat with Mom, for Carol's Christmas catalogs and the wonderful dreams about Christmas future, for a day to putter in my room, for the chance to watch Becky eat cotton candy, for our tucking-in routine that brings comfort to Mom and me. Love, Sue

OCTOBER 15, 2001

Yesterday was a fair day for Mom. She slept till 9 when I woke her, so she could take her pain medicine. Around 10:30 I fixed some breakfast for us. Shortly afterwards, Mom had an increase in pain and nausea. Uncle William and Aunt MM stopped by for a quick visit after church. I decided to fix a spaghetti sauce from scratch for dinner. Mom suggested I add two cloves to the sauce. It was just what it needed to make it wonderful. Mom slept from 3 till 6, when I woke her up for dinner. This is still a change from sleeping all day. We watched some TV and it was time for me to tuck her in and say our prayers. Mom appeared to sleep through the night.

Thank you God, for this day so sweet, for Sunday visits from Uncle William and Aunt MM and for Mom's help in making the spaghetti sauce. Love, Sue

OCTOBER 16, 2001

Yesterday was a good day for Mom. She was able to stay awake all day. I woke her at 9, so she could take her medicine and eat some toast. She said that she had slept well last night. I noticed Mom's right ear was bright red from laying on it all night. Fortunately the reddened area still blanches to touch. I told Mom that we would have to figure out something to protect her ear from developing a sore. She assured me that she knew that I would figure it out. Maybe I can fix some kind of foam cutout to protect her ear. After *The Price Is Right* Mom looked through Christmas catalogs.

I talked with Mom about having Carolyn increase her days from two to three days. It really is important that she have immaculate skin care. Mom said she was ok with that if I thought it was necessary. I also told her that I would be asking Kathy about the alternating pressure mattress for Mom's bed. It would really reduce her chances of developing a pressure sore. Mom took a walk around the house after lunch.

Kathy, the nurse, arrived shortly after Mom had gotten back in bed. She said she would take care of the pressure mattress. Mom is really warming up to her and that pleases me. Carolyn arrived at the end of Kathy's visit. Carolyn was agreeable to coming three times a week. We were surprised to find out that Susanne had mailed us a surprise Halloween package. Mom opened the package and found an orange plastic envelope filled with little candies and a book of postcards with photographs of cats. Mom also enjoyed reading her card from FiFi. After we ate dinner it was time for *The Antiques Roadshow* which we really enjoyed watching. After she finished reading her email I tucked her in and we said our prayers. She was up one time during the night.

When I went to let Grace out this morning, I was greeted with a 39° temperature. Grace and I were boogieing.

Thank you God, for this day so sweet, for a surprise package from Susanne, for *The Antiques Roadshow* and for Mom's confidence in my ability to care for her. Love, Sue

OCTOBER 18, 2001

Yesterday was a good day for Mom. She did have a couple of episodes of breakthrough pain. I suspect that it will soon be time to increase her routine, long acting oxycontin. She surprised me by asking for oatmeal for breakfast. It had been a long time since either of us has had oatmeal. I told Mom that the oatmeal had warmed my cockles. She just smiled and shook her head when I asked her what cockles were and did girls have them.

Mom watched her TV shows while I did some chores around the house. Marilyn called and wanted to come over and spend some time taping Mom, as she talked about her life memories. I decided to get out and run some errands. Lynda came a little after 3, to see Mom. Marilyn and Mom sat at the kitchen table, while Carolyn made Mom's bed. Marilyn needed to scoot and Lynda stayed with Mom till I got back from the store. I was pleased to find out that Mom had enjoyed herself while I was gone. Lynda told me, that she and Marilyn had talked about the hospital bed with Mom. I was comforted to find out that Mom feels like the hospital bed will be more comfortable than her own bed. The hospital bed will be delivered on Saturday.

Mom and I enjoyed our meatloaf dinner that Frances had prepared for us. We watched some TV and decided to turn in early. I tucked her in and we said our prayers. I was touched when I heard Mom giving thanks for being blessed with good friends. She slept through the night.

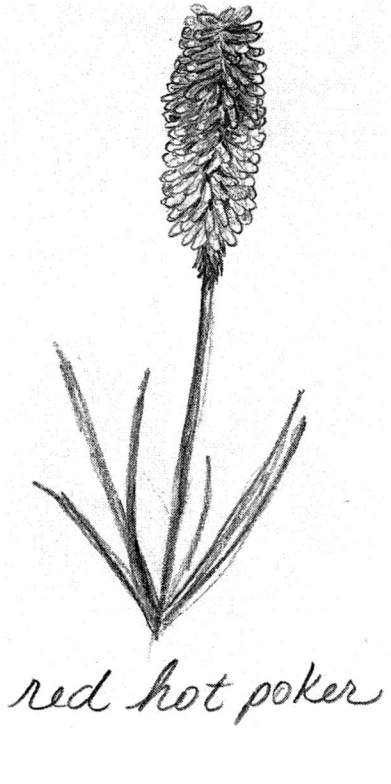

red hot poker

It was 47° when I let Grace out. I swear, if we had a lake outside our backdoor I would jump in the water and become a member of the polar bear club.

Thank you God, for this day so sweet, for wonderful oatmeal, for a glorious day to be out running errands and for Marilyn and Lynda who are beautiful examples of what friends are all about. Love, Sue

OCTOBER 19, 2001

Yesterday was a pretty good day for Mom. We started our day off with another bowl of oatmeal for breakfast. Mom told me that she wanted to make a suggestion. She wants me to get out one day a week, at least, and with some help from who was staying with her, she wants to prepare a meal. I was very pleased to hear that she felt strong enough to attempt to cook a meal. After lunch she walked to the front porch to check out how the resodding of grass in the front yard looked. We sat on the front porch and took in the beautiful weather. Kathy came shortly after we came back in the house. When we were alone, she acknowledged my mixed feelings about the hospital bed. Mother is firmly in favor of making the change.

I spent some time watering in the afternoon. I am amazed at how beautiful most of Mom's flowers still are at the end of October. I came in to prepare dinner and thought I would prepare a new recipe. I made pan fried squash patties. They were wonderful with Becky's beef derrington. Mom got nauseated right as I served her dinner. I told her that a compazine would calm things down and I could reheat her dinner. We watched *Who Wants to be a Millionaire* and then turned in for the night. Mom appears to have slept through the night.

Thank you God, for this day so sweet, for green grass and for Mom's new goals. Love, Sue

OCTOBER 20, 2001

Mom and I had a wonderful day yesterday. We started getting ready to go to the beauty shop. Mom was going to have a haircut, style, manicure and pedicure and I was going to have a pedicure. Before we left for the beauty shop, Fausto, our volunteer, came by so I could show him how I water Mom's garden. He really is a terrific young man. Bryant stopped by as we were walking out the door. He helped Mom into the car and off we went. It was a beautiful day to be driving. When we got to the beauty shop they treated Mom like a queen. There were pillows behind her and under her as she sat getting her hair and nails done. As we were leaving, Maria, her beautician, told Mom that if she could not make it in, she would come to the house and give her a haircut. We were both touched by how kind everyone was.

I stopped by this deli that we like and picked up some chicken wrap sandwiches and soup for later. It was 3:30 and neither one of us had eaten lunch. We ate our sandwiches as we drove. Before we got home Mom wanted to stop and get a basket for her walker. I was surprised when I was ready to head home, with basket in hand, she wanted to go to Eckerds and pick out some nail polish. Mom has not been in a store shopping since the first of August. We finished up and headed home. What a wonderful word home is to all of us that are blessed to have a home. We finished dinner and were treated to the show *America's Funniest Videos*. Mom and I both laughed out loud at some of the videos we saw. What a wonderful end to a full day.

I tucked her in and we said our prayers. Mom appears to have slept all night. Today is the day that they deliver the hospital bed.

Thank you God, for this day so sweet, for seeing Mom dressed in her beautiful clothes, for the tender care that was so freely offered at the beauty shop, for the opportunity to go shopping with Mom and for the shared belly laughs. Love, Sue

OCTOBER 21, 2001

Yesterday was a nice day for Mom. She hit a couple of rough patches with pain, but she responded well to her PRN pain medicines. I took a few pictures of her in her big bed. I knew that I would never see her in that bed again. I had already talked with Mom about my feelings about her bed, so I decided not to continue to process my sadness about her moving from her bed to a hospital bed. The move was critical for her comfort and her skin integrity. I presented a positive attitude about the many benefits of her new bed. I remember a very wise person's advice about changes…"If you can't change your circumstances, you can change your attitude about your circumstances." I actively practice that advice in my life.

Becky, Tom and Sherri got here before the hospital bed was

delivered. In the process of cleaning out from underneath the bed, Tom called to me and told me that Mom needed me. When I got to the room Mom was on the floor and everyone was standing around her. She had a big "I gotcha" grin on her face. She had told me earlier in the morning that she had a big surprise planned for me. I told Mom and the whole group of them that I was going to tell my big sister on them. Mom just laughed and continued pulling out the card table from under the bed. The practical joke and the subsequent laughter was most welcomed by me. Mom planned this out, to relieve the sadness of closing this part of her life. All of this made me question if Mom really was going through a detachment phase. Maybe a couple of weeks ago Mom was sleeping a lot of the time because of the medicine. I certainly will not forget that mischievous glimmer in her eyes when I discovered her on the floor. The hospital bed got set up and Becky and I found some pretty sheets for it. We also picked out this beautiful blue quilt with stars on it for Mom's bed. She told us that she had pieced that quilt in the summer of her tenth year. I can't imagine being ten years old and doing that kind of quality of handwork. It was a nice day with everybody working together with the goal of making Mom feel happy and secure, and also have her home and garden be pleasing and a comfort to her. Becky and Tom certainly excel at doing that every Saturday.

After they left for the day, Mom read her email and her mail. She also felt up to making some phone calls to friends and family. Mom's voice has really not recovered fully since her surgery in July. She has avoided, at times, talking on the phone because it causes her to strain her voice so she can be heard.

We had Becky's King Ranch Chicken Casserole for dinner. Mom really enjoyed it and cleaned her plate. In our prayers, Mom thanked God for the many blessings she has received from her friends, her family and her faith. It was a 2-honk night. Mom is sleeping in this morning. We will have brunch when she wakes up.

Thank you God, for this day so sweet, for the freedom to choose how we deal with what life brings to us, for Mom's being playful to make this transition easier, for the sparkle in her eyes, for the sweet discovery of her childhood quilt, for Becky's casserole and for our shared nightly prayers. Love, Sue

OCTOBER 22, 2001

Mom had a so-so day yesterday. I woke her at 10 so she could take her medicine and get her day started. I scrambled eggs with green chilies and onion. Mom cleaned her plate. She was having some significant breakthrough pain, so she had to take extra pain medicine. I read the Sunday paper and she dozed till 1:30. Uncle William and Aunt MM stopped by for a short visit. After they left, Mom ate some lunch. About an hour later she began vomiting. I have a routine that I do with her meds, shaved ice and a cold cloth, that seems to get things under control and Mom is comforted with our routine. I knew that the combination of pain and nausea medications would make her sleepy.

While Mom was sleeping I called Diane to vent a little bit. I was concerned that Mom is choosing to stay in an upright position in bed, even when she slept last night. I have tried to tell her that she needs to change from side to side in bed. In fact, after I medicated her for nausea and pain, I suggested that she turn on her left side. She muttered under her breath, "I know, Sue, I will do it later." I am choosing to tell myself that it is the medication impacting her judgment and I am also going to tell Kathy on her. Kathy can play the bad guy. Having the nurse play the bad guy is one of the reasons I wanted hospice. I knew there would be times that I would have trouble being firm about certain aspects of her care. I wanted to be in the position to give comfort during the hard parts. Diane and I also talked about the stress at her job and Gordon's daily 4:30 a.m. concerns that the world was coming to an end because of the flooding. Diane laughed when I told her that

I felt a lot better about my situation, after hearing about her situation. If you can laugh about it, "it" can't get you.

I woke Mom at 6:30 p.m., so she could eat and take her scheduled pain medications. After we ate dinner, Mom was still very groggy and she wanted to go back to sleep. I was surprised when she agreed to lower her head and lay on her left side, with a pillow behind her back. She remained on her side through the night. I wasn't so concerned about turning her because of the alternating air pressure mattress.

Mom woke at 4:30, complaining of a severe sore throat. I got her some lozenges and made a cup of hot chocolate. She seemed comforted by this, so I returned to bed. It had been a 3-honk night.

Thank you God, for this day so sweet, for scrambled eggs with green chilies and onions, for the Sunday morning paper, for the Gaither Gospel Hour, for sisters that you can always laugh with and for hot chocolate. Love, Sue

OCTOBER 23, 2001

Mom had a hard time with pain, sore throat and nausea yesterday. She is having to take her medicine for breakthrough pain more frequently. I will talk to Kathy about increasing her routine pain medicine. I don't know what this sore throat is all about. It could be just a plain old sore throat.

My friend Gail was able to come to the house and get a pulse oximeter reading on me, so that Medicare would start paying for my oxygen and I could start using liquid oxygen again. This reading is the oxygen saturation level in my blood. I had to have a reading done while I was off oxygen and it could not be any higher than 89%. All that is involved is they put this little clip on a finger and it can tell what your saturation level is. My level was 84%, so I passed or failed depending on how you look at it. Gail coming to the house saved me a lot of time sitting and waiting and waiting in my pulmonologists office.

Mom decided to have some of Marilyn's vegetable soup for lunch. I had some of her soup in the freezer for this kind of day. Mom and I talked about her cooking while I was at the doctor's office on Tuesday. I am not sick. It is a routine visit, so I can get my prescriptions renewed. She expressed some doubt as to whether she would be feeling like cooking after having such a rough day. I told her that there were no deadlines involved with when she decided to cook. Marianne, the social worker, came and spent some time talking with me. She was stressing how important it is to get out of the house. She spoke to me about Mom probably struggling with increased weakness and losing some of the power to control things in her life. It would be hard for anyone to have to depend on someone else's help in the bathroom, with very personal tasks. It is so good to have someone that is not family give feedback on their observations. Mom did not feel up to talking because of her throat.

After Carolyn and Mariann left, Mom caught up on reading her emails. Aunt MM called to tell me that she could stay with Mom while I was at the doctor's office. Mom enjoys Mary Margaret and is looking forward to their visit. I started putting dinner together. We had Becky's special meatloaf, mashed potatoes, peas and frozen cranberry salad. Mom and I watched *The Antique Roadshow*. We said our prayers and it was time for bed. Mom honked once during the night.

Thank you God, for this day so sweet, for my friend Gail, who made my life less complicated, for Marilyn's vegetable soup and for your love that is made tangible through our friends and family. Love, Sue

Frozen Cranberry Salad

2 3-oz. packages cream cheese

2 Tbs sugar

2 Tbs mayonnaise

1 16 oz. can whole jellied cranberry sauce

1 8-oz. can crushed pineapple

½ cup chopped pecans

1 cup whipping cream

½ cup powdered sugar

1 tsp vanilla extract

    Combine first three ingredients, stirring till smooth

    Stir in cranberry sauce, pineapple and pecans

    Beat whipping cream till foamy

    Gradually add powdered sugar, beating until smooth

    Stir in vanilla

    Fold whipped cream mixture into cranberry mixture

    Spoon into 8 inch square dish

    Cover and freeze till firm

    Cut into squares

    Makes 9 servings

OCTOBER 24, 2001

Mom had a fair day yesterday. She had two rough patches with pain that responded quickly to her pain medicine. She admitted being anxious about me leaving the house to go to the doctor. Aunt MM was going to stay with her while I was gone. Before I left to go to the doctor, I told Mom that I should be back around 3. I was not sure about how long I would be kept waiting. I was kept waiting and did not get home till 10 after 3. Mom looked at me and said, "Where were you, I was getting scared. You said you would be home by 3." I took her to the bathroom and found out that she had called Becky in a panic about my whereabouts. She did not tell Becky that she was scared to walk with Aunt MM and needed to go to the bathroom. She told me that she knew I needed to get out, but she really only felt safe with me. I told her that I would not have left her with anyone that could not help her. I felt a little helpless. I guess I will need to give Mom more reassurance that the friends and family that stay with her can help her with any problem that may arise.

While I was gone Janet, the chaplain, came by for a visit. She is very comforting to be around. Kathy, the nurse, came by shortly after I got back home. I need to say again how much I like her and feel comforted that she is my mother's nurse. I am so happy that I spoke up and did not just settle for the first nurse that Mom was assigned. Kathy was not pleased with the kind of mattress that was delivered to Mom, so she called and arranged for a better air mattress. Kathy had shared her email address with me. I laughed when she said her address was kind of strange. I asked her if it was stranger than nosewhistler. She laughed and said hers was nursiwursi. One more time, I really like Mom's nurse, Kathy.

Mom and I had a relaxed dinner and watched *Unsolved Mysteries*. Before she turned in for the night, Mom read her email from Jenny. It was such a sweet note. She faithfully writes a note every morning. It was a 1-honk night. Mom was still asleep at 8. Grace and I are waiting for a cool front to move in.

Thank you God, for this day so sweet, for Aunt MM's help, for a nurse with an email address nursiwursi and for Jenny's faithful notes every morning. Love, Sue

OCTOBER 25, 2001

Mom had a nice day yesterday. We were surprised when a new aid named Vicky showed up at our door. Heartland did not call us and let us know that Carolyn was not coming back. Vicky seems very friendly and Mom seemed to enjoy the attention. After Vicky left, they came to deliver Mom's new flotation air mattress. After the mattress was set up Becky arrived, bearing fried chicken for Mom's lunch. Becky had taken some time away from her office to clean out the attic. She never ceases to amaze me. Of course, we had our routine…Becky finds a bug…Becky throws the bug on Sue…Sue screams…Becky smiles. We can now finish the task at hand, since we have completed our ages old ritual…"Lets see how loud I can make Sue scream, with this big nasty looking bug." I wouldn't tell Becky, but there is something comforting about how some things don't change between sisters.

Mom took a short nap while Becky was up in that hot dusty attic making it less dusty and more organized. Mom woke up and decided to try her hand at a few recipes that are favorites. Becky and I were happy to see Mom in the kitchen. She had plans of making beef and beans and Ekridge sausage, rice and Rotel tomatoes. They were both real easy meals to put together. Becky had to leave while we were still in the kitchen. I took pictures of Mom cooking to help preserve this memory. Mom read her emails after she returned to bed. She enjoys reading Jenny's daily notes and was pleased when I gave her an email card from Margie that I had printed out. Margie is a childhood friend of Mom's. I think it is so wonderful that they are still in touch. Mom took a nap until it was time for dinner. It was a special dinner as far as I was concerned. I was not expecting to ever have the opportunity to eat another meal that Mom had cooked. I froze part of each meal, so when Diane comes she can have some of Mom's home cooking. We watched a show on flea market finds and decided to call it a night.

I was so comforted by our prayers last night. I was surprised to find Mom hurting at 2:30 when she honked for me. She usually is comfortable at night. I gave her the extra oxycontin with ice water and tucked her in extra tight. Before I returned to bed, I said a prayer that Mom would soon feel comfortable. She grabbed my hand and told me that she was going to be ok and I could rest easy.

I was very pleased to find the temperature to be 42°. I did a kind of a Chuck Berry "step and scoot." I swear I heard the cats asking Grace how long winter lasted and Grace told them that, in dog years, a very long time.

Thank you God, for this day so sweet, for the gift of watching Mom cook some old favorites, for baby sisters, for Margie, a life long friend, and for the peace that comes with prayer. Love, Sue

OCTOBER 26, 2001

Mom had a nice day yesterday. She asked for oatmeal for breakfast. Mom likes it cooked with milk. Mom commented how nice it was to have breakfast with me and I readily agreed. I went on and printed out her morning email. She was so pleased to find, in addition to Jenny's morning note and a funny note from Diane, Debi had written a sweet note.

Marilyn called to tell me that she was coming over around 1 p.m. to visit with Mom. She suggested that I take that time and get out for a while. It sounded good to me, since I needed to pick up some prescriptions and a few other things. When I told Mom about Marilyn coming she was excited at the prospect of a visit from Marilyn, but got anxious at the idea of me leaving the house. She was afraid I would not be there if she had some kind of pain, nausea or bathroom emergency. I reminded her that Marilyn had stayed with her all day when I went to the fair. She said that she knew that and she knew I needed to get out, but it scared her. I spent a little time talking with her about what we could do to help her feel safe. Mom will have to find a way to be comforted by others that are helping care for her. There will be times that I have to get away from the house. She does know that her fears are not rational and I have to leave the house for different reasons.

Marilyn arrived bearing gifts of photographs of Mom and Frances and a small basket with miniature corn, squash and pumpkins. She even took a picture of Mom and me sitting on the side of her bed. It did not look like I was going to get to leave. I was waiting for my oxygen guy to deliver my liquid oxygen. I could not leave until we had switched out my concentrator for the tall tanks of liquid oxygen. I felt like I was waiting for Christmas to arrive. The liquid oxygen is a fraction more pure and it is so much easier on my nose, plus it comes with a little oxygen tank you can wear like a fanny pack. I fill my little tank off of the big tanks and it gives me a lot more control with how much oxygen I have available to me when I need to leave the house. He finally came and Marilyn said she could stay with Mom till I got back from the store.

When I returned, Marilyn said that they had talked about recipes while I was gone. Mom said she had done ok and was happy that I had a chance to get out of the house. Mom took a short nap while I did some chores around the house. We had the sausage and rice she had prepared for dinner. She seemed to take pleasure in eating a meal she had cooked. I know that I certainly did. After we had watched some TV, we said our prayers and turned in for the night. Mom woke at 3 and needed to go to the bathroom. I got her settled back in bed and returned to my bed. It was not an hour later when the whole house was startled awake by the house alarm going whoop-whoop. There is a speaker in the hall where the alarm company can speak to us to assess what the problem is. You have to remember the password or he will send out the police. He told me that the alarm was coming from the panic button. I told him no one was pressing any button. He suggested that the battery might be low. Before I could get the battery out, he had signed off and the alarm came back on. It is a very loud alarm. I tried to get him back on the speaker, but he was gone. I realized that Mom had always taken care of everything involving the alarm system. I asked her if she could remember the security pin number. She said it had been too long since she had used it. The alarm is still screaming and I cannot find the phone number to the security company. I decide to go to the keypad and clear my head and see if I can come up with the code spontaneously. This will make Diane crazy, but I typed in the right code. I don't know where it came from, but the alarm turned off. I am going to locate the security company's phone number and pin it on my bulletin board. I was wide awake, but decided to go on and lay down for a while.

Mom honked at 6 and wanted to eat. I decided that even though the day had started at 3 it was a good sign that Mom was hungry.

Thank you God, for this day so sweet, for surprise emails from Debi, for Marilyn's generous spirit, for liquid oxygen and for the gift of a meal prepared by my mother. Love, Sue

OCTOBER 27, 2001

Mom had a pretty good day yesterday. Kathy, Mom's nurse, arrived fairly early in the morning. She spent some time just chatting with Mom. They were talking about painting rooms and she was complementing Mom on how comfortable her house felt. Mom was just beaming after their chat. While Kathy was still here, Vicky, the new aide, arrived. Vicky has the most incredible East Texas accent. When she calls Mom "honey" (pretty close to sugar) or says "bless your heart," it is like it wraps you up in a homemade quilt stitched with love and faith. I had Vicky put Mom's flannel sheets on her bed. Kathy and Vicky had a fit over them. The sheets have dogs and cats on them and they are all holding umbrellas like it is raining cats and dogs. I told them that Becky had found those sheets for Mom. Becky thought the sheets would provide extra warmth and extra smiles. Vicky told Mom that there was no doubt in her mind of how much her children love her.

After Kathy and Vicky left, Mom told me that she had been given the best bath that she could remember receiving. Kathy and Vicky

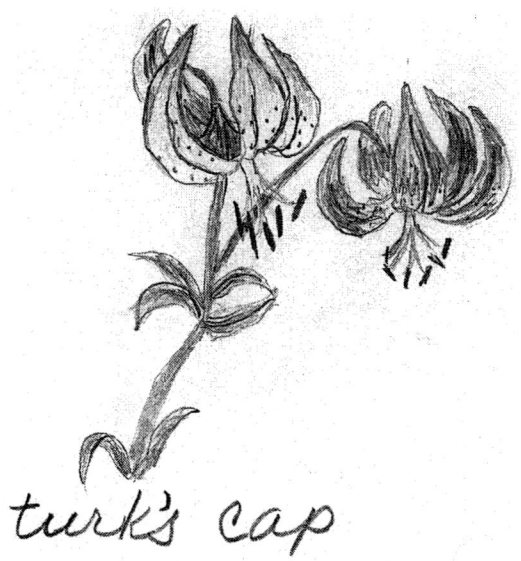

turk's cap

really give the kind of care anyone would want for their own mom. I have been able to let go of this "I'm on guard stance," when they are around.

After Mom had lunch, Fausto, our volunteer, arrived to water Mom's garden. He is taking a piano course in college. I had asked him to bring his music, so he could practice. Mom and I were pleased to hear him practice his music. After he had watered the garden and had practiced the piano for a while, he questioned Mom in some detail about the stories behind the pictures in her room. Mom showed him her Halloween costume and her smile on a stick. I wrote earlier about her costume being these purple glasses with bushy pink eyebrows attached to the glasses, along with a huge green witch's nose with warts and complete with snaggleteeth. Her smile on a stick is a big cardboard grin on a stick. Mom will whip out that smile and plop it under her nose when she thinks I could use an extra special smile. Fausto got a big kick out of Mom's style show.

After he left, we spent some time looking at catalogs and talking about Christmas. I wish I could have bottled how sweet that afternoon felt. I know that the memory will bring a lot of comfort for future times. Mom hit a rough spot after dinner. She became nauseated and started to vomit. I had to add an extra Ativan to our routine to get things under control. I knew that Mom would get extra sleepy. It was close enough to bedtime, so I said our prayers and tucked her in for the night.

We had a 2-honk night. It was 42° again this morning. I danced a little modified pony step. There were no comments from the gallery. Their silence did speak volumes about their attitude regarding spontaneous cold weather dancing. The cats left the room when I broke into song. I had to sing *Happy Birthday* to Grace. This is her thirteenth birthday. I can't begin to find words to describe how I feel about her love, faithful companionship, not to mention her role as Mom's night nurse that she has blessed me with. I was so blessed when Grace came into my life.

Thank you God, for this day so sweet, for Vicky and her comforting voice and words, for the piano music Fausto shared with us, for the incredible joy, peace and comfort that Grace has brought to the last thirteen years of my life. Love, Sue (a grateful friend to "Amazing Grace The Wonder Dog." That is her birth name.)

OCTOBER 28, 2001

Mom had a long, hard day yesterday. I have questioned whether I should write about yesterday. I want to protect Mom. I don't want to acknowledge this part of Mom's end of life journey. I started writing so I could include Diane in on what was happening to her mother as she comes to the end of her life and my role as her daughter and primary care giver. When I went to wake up Mom, it smelled like she had had an accident. She denied needing to go to the bathroom. What she wanted the most was to eat some cereal. I pretended to convince myself that it was probably just gas. After she ate her cereal, she finally agreed to go to the bathroom. I felt so sad for Mom when it became obvious that she had had an accident. She looked so totally defeated. I reminded her that she had to take extra medicine last night for nausea and pain and that was probably why she had an accident. She and I both were quiet as I helped her to get cleaned up. I am so sorry now that I had been so vocal about not being able to cope with patients that had pooped. My line was, "I am a psychiatric nurse and I only deal with the neck up problems. I don't do poop." That comment must be running through her head. My guess would be that she is horrified at having to depend on me for assistance with such an intimate task. I told her that I was surprised to find out that I had been wrong all these years, because I had not forgotten how to be an all-purpose nurse like Pernell was. (Pernell was the male nurse that worked with me and dealt with all the problems associated with incontinence).

Shortly after I got Mom settled into bed, Becky and Tom arrived. Mom immediately told Becky that she had to get to the bathroom. Mom was not able to make it to the bathroom in time. Becky assisted Mom in getting cleaned up. When Becky came out of the bathroom and saw how sad I looked, she made a funny face at me. Becky was not only taking care of Mom, but was taking care of me. Becky is certainly not immune to the feelings of sadness when she sees her mother struggling to maintain some dignity, privacy and control of her body. Before Becky had gotten Mom tucked in bed, Mom told her she needed to hurry back to the bathroom. Again it was too late. Becky helped Mom get cleaned up and again made funny faces at me. I had tears in my eyes as I watched all this happen.

After Becky had tucked Mom in bed, she went back to the bathroom to finish cleaning up. I walked in and gave her a big hug. I told her "thank you" for stepping in with Mom and the funny faces for me. I was overwhelmed with gratitude for having been blessed with a sister named Becky. Mom was so exhausted with all the trips to the bathroom that she was asleep in no time.

Lynda arrived. We were going to get out and do some poking around. Becky, Tom, Lynda and I visited for quite a while in the kitchen. We were complimenting Tom for his many talents to build and repair things around the house. He was in the process of putting together a cabinet for Mom's bathroom. Mom really does love him as a son and is so grateful for all the help he has been in maintaining her home. Lynda and I went and had lunch at Chilis. She was so supportive as I talked about the mixture of feelings I had in regards to Mom's recent loss of bowel control. I am angry that she is having to endure this indignity. I am sad, as well, that she is having to endure this indignity. I am standing on the sidelines as I watch my Mother's body betray her and I can't prevent it from happening. I remind myself that God tells us to find joy in all that we do. I will have to work on that one.

While we were out, Lynda and I went to a bicycle shop to get a bell for Mom's walker. Instead of a bell we found a wondrous bright green frog horn that we can clamp on her walker. I decided that she needed something to make the animals move into the slow lane while she is navigating down the hall to the bathroom. I also had decided that Mom's basket on her walker was screaming to be decorated. We went to a party store to look for a patriotic flag and a Halloween decoration for the grill work on her basket. We did not find a flag, but I found a big ugly purple and black spider with piercing red eyes. I knew that Becky would be so impressed with my plans to decorate Mom's walker.

When we got home, Becky told me that Mom woke up from her nap and realized that she had yet had another accident. I focused on getting Mom's walker decorated. Tom put the frog horn on Mom's walker and Becky really gave the horn a workout. She was speechless when she saw the big-ass, red-eyed, ugly spider. I am sure she was impressed with how tasteful it was, not to mention how useful it will be.

After they left, Lynda stayed a while to visit with Mom. I was pleased to see Mom clean her dinner plate. Lynda was headed home when Bryant stopped by to visit with Mom. While he was here Mom expelled some gas and I asked her, if she wanted to go to the bathroom. She initially declined, but after I insisted she complied with my request. As it turns out, she had another accident. Mom told me that she was concerned that she was having trouble making it to the bathroom in time. I told her we could talk to Kathy about it on Tuesday when she came to assess Mom. I truly don't know what to think. Mom has had accidents in the past, but nothing like this. I know it is not uncommon for people that are dying to become incontinent. It was not supposed to happen to my Mother.

I tucked her in extra tight after we said our prayers. I woke at 4 and found Mom awake. She said that she had just returned to bed after going to the bathroom. She said she was just barely able to avoid another accident. I tucked her in again and returned to bed. I ended up not going back to sleep.

When I let Grace out the temperature was 45°. This morning I celebrated with a little cha-cha-cha. The cats turned their back to me. I heard Ringo tell Max not to look because it only encourages her. Cold temperatures are what inspire me.

Thank you God, for this day so sweet, for the gift of Becky's comfort and support, for the joy of finding out that I really am able to be an all-purpose nurse/daughter in providing care for my mother, for Tom's faithful help in maintaining a safe and comfortable home for Mom and me, for a magical bright green frog horn, for the long talk over lunch with Lynda and for Diane's words of comfort and support last night. Love, Sue

OCTOBER 29, 2001

Yesterday was filled with "remember when" conversations with her sister FiFi, nephew Stephen, older brother William and sister-in-law Mary Margaret. Our day started fairly early since we set our clocks back one hour. The clock said 6, but our body said 7. Mom and I were so excited about the company we were about to have. She got up and freshened up. Mom wanted to know if we had any cookies we could serve with the coffee. I had something better-French Silk Pie.

Aunt FiFi and Stephen arrived around 10:30 a.m. Stephen had brought his camera to capture some of the day on film. Uncle Dade had stayed home this time with his care giver. He is as frail as Mom and I am sure he appreciated being able to stay in the comfort of his home. He was missed though. In the past, Uncle Dade always had a smile and wonderful stories to tell. Stephen and I had a chance to visit alone while FiFi, William and MM visited with Mom. We talked about our involvement in our parents care. Uncle Dade can sleep 20 or so hours a day, like Mom was doing a while back. Stephen also talked about the difficulty in understanding much of his Dad's speech. He told me that he could really identify with missing my mom. We also talked about being in the position of helping our parent, after they have had an accident. Stephen shared some helpful hints that made things easier when faced with this task. Our situations with our parent are so very similar. Uncle Dade is 91½ years old and his health has been failing. We both also feel like we have a bank of wonderful memories of time spent with our parents. It felt so comforting to talk with Stephen. He has a wonderfully warm, soft voice. I am so happy that I have a cousin like Stephen to share this part of our lives together. He and Susanne have to travel thousands of miles to come home to see their parents. They always include as many visits as possible to Dallas to visit with us. It would be so easy to find reasons not to come for a visit. I know we were all brought up with the same conviction of how blessed we were to have a family and how important it was not to miss out on opportunities to spend time with family.

FiFi and William seemed to really enjoy their "remember when" stories. At one point, everybody went outside to enjoy the many butterflies in Mom's garden. Her garden is still blooming. It is full of birds and butterflies. The visit came to an end too soon, but Mom was getting tired. I felt like I was walking on clouds when Uncle William and Aunt FiFi complemented me on how I was caring for Mom. Aunt FiFi said that she wished she could be closer and more involved. I told her that her daily notes were a very important part of our everyday routine. Jenny is writing daily notes to her Granny because of the example that Aunt FiFi set. This certainly shows how you can still be involved on a daily basis, even if you live far away. It would be a mistake to ever take your family for granted. Without family, caring for Mom would be impossible.

After they left for home, Mom took a short nap while I finished pulling dinner together. We were going to have a bonafide Sunday dinner of roast, mashed potatoes, pan fried squash patties and spiced apple rings. Before Mom could start eating, she became nauseated and began to throw up. Things eventually calmed down, but she did not feel like she could eat. I assured her that it did not hurt my feelings. I made her promise me that if she got hungry she would honk for me. I did leave some goldfish crackers at her bedside, just in case.

We said our prayers and I tucked her in tight for the night. It was a 2-honk night. She had attempted to go to the bathroom on her own and had gotten her walker turned around backwards. She used her green frog horn to let me know that she needed help. See Becky-it turned out to be a very useful addition to her walker.

When I let Grace out, the temperature was 47°. I felt somewhat subdued, so I did a little 1-2-3 waltz step. Cats can be so critical. I heard Ringo tell Max that I was no Ginger Rogers.

Thank you God, for this day so sweet, for a cousin named Stephen, for Aunt FiFi's love and loyalty to her baby sister, for the beauty of Mom's garden and for a green frog horn that came to Mom's rescue. Love, Sue

OCTOBER 30, 2001

Yesterday was an extremely hard day for Mom. Before Vicky came, she had two accidents. When Vicky got here to help Mom with her bath she had two more major accidents. Lynda stopped by for a visit with Mom. While she was here, Mom had seven accidents. Lynda stepped up to the plate and helped Mom with all seven accidents. At one point, Mom busted out crying. She told me she was so sorry that we were having to deal with all of these accidents. I sat there and patted her leg and Lynda told her that this was not a problem for her, that she knew she was embarrassed, but she couldn't have picked two people more equipped to deal with such situations. Mom turned and looked at me. I reminded her that I had returned to my all-purpose nursing mind set, and that I felt so sad she was having to experience this, but the silver lining in all this is that I can handle it without any emergency evacuations. She smiled and told me that she had noticed that I had been very calm during all of this. We were trying to figure out what in the world was going on in Mom's gut. One of my guesses would have been that she had just returned from vacation from a third world country with a questionable water supply. We will certainly discuss all of this with Kathy.

Mom said she was hungry for some popcorn chicken. Lynda hopped right on that and went and got her lunch. I gave her a second Immodium with her lunch. While Mom was resting, Lynda and I talked about what was going on with Mom. I was at a loss for words to thank her for all of her help. She reminded me that she had told me from the very beginning of Mom's illness she would be walking right beside me. She also told me that it was important to her to have a chance to help Mom, whatever the problem might be. I know that Mom was extremely comforted to have Lynda by her side as she was confronted with having to deal with all the insults of all the accidents.

Mom was able to take a short nap before dinner. When she woke up, she said she was hungry for roast and gravy. Unfortunately, Mom had another accident. We quickly dealt with it and I gave her a third Immodium. We were able to watch *The Antique Roadshow* without incident. After the show Mom looked startled and told me "let's go." She almost made it to the bathroom. She commented on how she had succeeded in stinking up the house. I told her, as far as I was concerned, I smelled an acute gastritis-like illness. I did not want her to paint herself as a slob or someone that was rude. I reminded her that she needed to be extra nice to herself, especially with her having to deal with such an acute illness. She did tell me that I was right. I also encouraged her to truly accept what Lynda and I told her about how fortunate we all were, because we were well equipped to deal with any emergency. She smiled real big and gave me a big kiss. I felt it important to not gloss over what happened with Mom today. To feel betrayed by your body and also be dependent on others to help you with very personal tasks of cleaning your body is something we all pray will not happen to us or someone we love. The fact is, when you are dying, you will probably be faced with many betrayals of your body. I wanted to let all of you know how it is being dealt with in this house.

Mom had a 2-honk night and one small accident. Just maybe, things are beginning to slow down.

It was 40° when I let Grace out. She was not a very enthusiastic participant in a little bunny hop step. I know Grace is saving up for when it really gets cold. I overheard Ringo tell Max to be thankful that they had not been forced into being a part of the bunny hop line.

Thank you God, for this day so sweet, for the blessing of Lynda and her wonderful nurturing ways, for the tears Mom shared with Lynda and I and for the gift of Immodium. Love, Sue

OCTOBER 31, 2001

Mom had a much easier day yesterday. There was just one very early morning accident. We started the day almost tip toeing, so we didn't stir anything up. Mom chose to have toast for breakfast, because toast has a reputation of being safe. Uncle William and Aunt MM came by for a visit. I was surprised at how verbal Mom was, when describing how hard a day yesterday was for her. She said that she was so thankful that Lynda and I helped her through a nightmare day. Uncle William surprised me with a big hug as he was walking to the front door. As he patted my back, I noticed that his eyes were full of tears. He thanked me for taking such good care of his sister. I told him I was so thankful to have the chance to be at my mother's side as she finishes the last part of her journey home.

After they left, Kathy arrived to assess Mom. Mom was pleased to see Kathy and talked to her about how hard yesterday was for her. She also delighted in pointing out her walker and the green frog horn, not to mention her big black spider that is attached to her basket. Kathy was impressed with the flannel sheep sheets that Becky gave Mom. Mom just glowed when Kathy told her that she must be the most loved mother in the world. Have I mentioned how much I like her as Mom's nurse? I am so glad that we spoke up and got a change of nurses.

Mom was able to clean her plate at lunch without there being any problems with her tummy. We are still tip toeing through this day. I started to prepare our dinner. I decided we would have pork chops cooked in the crock pot, beets, purple hull peas and new potatoes. Mom and I had discussed the menu and felt we would be safe with what I was cooking. Mom took a long nap before dinner. I know she was so afraid that she was going to have a repeat of yesterday.

I talked with Becky about the problem with Mom's mattress pad. Kathy had told us that the heated mattress pad on Mom's bed was probably not letting the flotation mattress perform at it s best. True to form, Becky got right on it and picked up an electric blanket to keep Mom warm. I woke Mom so she could eat her dinner and read her email and her regular mail. After dinner, Kelly and Lynda came over. Lynda was going to stay with Mom while Kelley took me to this house in Garland that is totally decorated with everything Halloween. What a wonderful treat to have a chance to see a home where folks don't hide their enthusiasm for holidays. They had a huge inflated black spider on the roof. There were big ghosts and little ghosts, witches with boiling cauldrons and skeletons that rolled their eyes and chattered their teeth, not to mention the fog machine and the music that was playing. There is no way I could fit all that we saw in this note, but trust me-it was magical. I know one thing for sure. I would like to meet the homeowners that could create such magic.

When we got home Mom listened intently as I described our adventure. Kelley got to telling stories, as only she can, complete with accents and gestures that made you feel that you were smack dab in the middle of the story. All we could do was laugh and laugh.

After they left for home, I walked Mom to the bathroom. When she pulled her panties down she said, "Ta-Dah." I fell out laughing. She was so excited that she still had not had any accidents. When she went "Ta-Dah", I was looking for a rabbit, because that is what magicians say when they pull a bunny out of their hat. I was so happy for Mom and her magic panties.

After our prayers, I tucked her in tight. We had a 1-honk night.

It was 51° when I let Grace outside. I told the cats that they were off the hook this time because I don't get inspired at 51°.

Thank you God, for this day so sweet, for Uncle William's hug, for flannel sheets with sheep on them, for those wonderful folks and their magic Halloween house, for the gift of Kelley's stories and how they transport you to another place and time and for my Mom's triumphant Ta-Dah! Love, Sue

NOVEMBER 1, 2001
Dria is the neighbor's three year old daughter

Mom had a pretty good day yesterday. She woke up hungry, so we had scrambled eggs and sausage. I told Mom that I had just gotten a call from an aide named Yolonda. She told me that Vickie was sick and would not be back. That was a real bummer to hear. Mom really liked Vicky. Yolonda told me that she could not be here until 4 p.m.

since she would be coming from her first job at UPS. I told her that we could try out that new time, but I was not sure it would work out. I will call Heartland tomorrow and find out what the deal is. I might find myself making noises of an unhappy customer concerning the frequent aide changes that Mom is having to experience. If I have to, I will have Becky call them. We really do need to feel like we feel safe with the team working with Mom and most importantly, that there is consistency of care. As a matter of fact, all Mom's children would take on anyone that could have a negative impact on her and her care. I know that as Mom's care giver, I have moved into a pseudo parental role with Mom. Fortunately, I still experience Mom's role as a parent. I savor the times when she questions whether I have gotten enough sleep or she fusses because I am not out playing more or the best feeling is when she gives me one of those "I know everything about you and I still love you" looks. I am painfully aware that will be the part of not having my mom physically present in my life that will be so desperately missed. My sisters and brother can give me a similar look, but it does not carry the same weight as one of Mom's "I know, love and treasure all that you are today and forever."

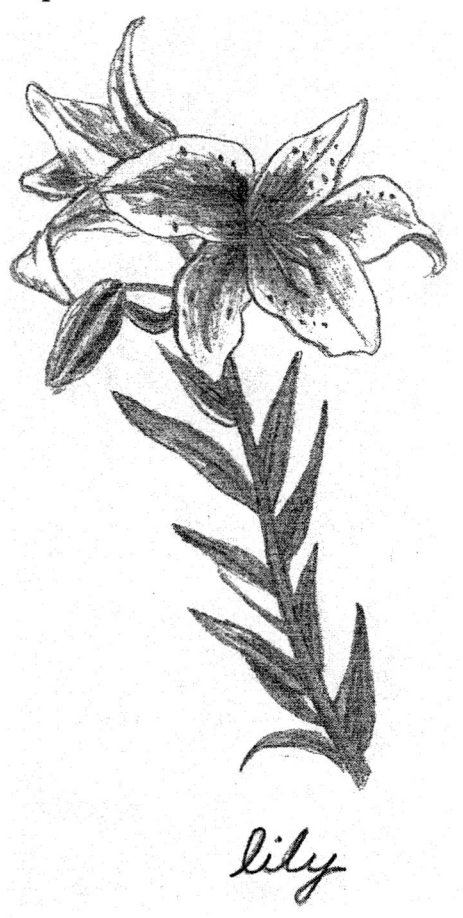

lily

In a situation of caring for a parent that is dying it is strange

104

how you can be in the role of parenting and your mom, with one look, reminds you that no matter what, she is still your mother. I am not ready to consider that there will be a time when the loving looks are gone in an instant. I savor and record in my memory each time Mom blesses me with one of her "looks."

Lynda came over in the afternoon, so I could get out and run a few errands. She also was planning on preparing a dinner of fried chicken and potato salad. Mom was excited about the dinner plans and truly seemed relaxed that Lynda would be staying with her. While I was out, I found some two inch thick foam that might work for Mom's ear that has a pressure sore. I want to cut the foam so it surrounds the outside of Mom's ear and protects the top of her ear from any pressure. I figure it will look kind of like a donut. I had to get a half of a yard so I have plenty of room for error.

When I returned home Lynda told me that Mom slept most of the time I was gone. When she did wake up, we went on and had a wonderful dinner. Lynda left shortly after dinner. Mom and I were waiting for a special visit from Dria. It wasn't long before Dria treated us to the vision of her dressed up as a Cinderella Princess. In Dria's words, she was a "Pincess." I got pictures of Mom and Dria together. What a wonderful visit from a little girl with a ponytail and a blue "Pincess" outfit, complete with shoes and crown.

Right after they left, Mom became extremely nauseated and threw up. I wish I knew what was behind these seemingly random episodes of nausea. Things calmed down and Mom and I said our prayers. It was a 1-honk night.

When I got up to let Grace out, it was 61°. Need I say more.

Thank you God, for this day so sweet, for Lynda's fried chicken, for a visit from a "Pincess" and for the look of enduring love in my Mother's eyes. Love, Sue

NOVEMBER 2, 2001

Mom had a nice day yesterday. I received a sad call from Margaret Ann. She called to tell me that our cousin Pat's husband had just died. I asked her how she was doing since her mother had died. She talked about how there had been some rough times, but she was healing. Her mother had lived with her and she was the primary care giver, like I am with Mom. Margaret Ann has been a wonderful source of comfort to me.

After breakfast, Janet, the chaplain, and Irene came by, at about the same time. Irene came bearing gifts of the last of the summer okra and a basket of persimmons. Janet found out that she went to school with Irene's children. It truly is a small world. I had told Janet about Mom's black Monday with all the accidents. She told me that she was sure that it was a difficult time for me to watch Mom decline. When she commented on how much Mom has declined since she first met her in August I was shocked to find myself wanting to give her a whack where her suspenders crossed. Her comment was accurate and meant to be supportive. I know that Mom has declined, but I guess I wasn't prepared to hear it confirmed out loud. I know that I have been writing about how weak, frail and dependent Mom has become, so where did all those defensive feelings come from? Before Janet made the comment about Mom declining, she had told me it was such a joy to visit us and see how much Mom and I enjoyed each other. Janet had lost her own mom when she was just 11 years old. In the past, she had told us that she would love to be a part of such a loving family. She also added how Mom was surrounded with her children, who knew without a doubt that they were loved by their mother. I guess her comment about Mom's decline was a sad reminder that Mom was really dying. I have moments where for maybe a short time I forget that Mom is dying. I guess I was relishing her observations on our loving relationships and it was a sudden painful reminder of the present reality of Mom's situation.

After they left, Mom lunched on Lynda's wonderful potato salad. It wasn't too long before she was sound asleep. While she was sleeping, I called the hospice to find out about Mom's status with her personal aide. It turns out that if we switched to Tuesday and Thursday, Vicky could still be our aide. I quickly agreed to that compromise. Mom was pleased to find out that she did not have to once again change aides. Mom ended up taking a long afternoon nap. When she woke later, she enjoyed reading her emails from Jenny, Marilyn and Cynthia.

It was a fairly quiet evening and Mom and I turned in early for the night. It was a 3-honk night.

When I went to let Grace out, I noticed that it was 61° outside. I asked Grace, "What's the use of going outside with it being so warm?" She was quick to point out there were other reasons to go out besides a cold temperature.

Thank you God, for this day so sweet, for the gift of Irene's home-grown persimmons, for a cousin named Margaret Ann and for the reminder of how blessed we are to have a mother that loved us and having the chance to show her how much we love her and cherish being able to care for her every need and desire. Love, Sue

NOVEMBER 3, 2001

Yesterday started out good and as the day progressed it got pretty rough for Mom. Mom was wanting to try to eat a bowl of oatmeal for breakfast. We were both concerned that the milk in the oatmeal might have contributed to her accidents on Monday. Mom is lactose intolerant. I told her if she was willing to give it a try, I would certainly prepare it for her. There did not seem to be any immediate consequence to the oatmeal. Kathy arrived as Mom was finishing her breakfast. Mom was telling Kathy that she and her mom had always had a lot of get up and go energy. Mom also added that of all her children, Becky seems to have inherited that energy. Kathy then encouraged Mom to talk about what it felt like to not feel like she has that energy to fall back on. Mom was able to talk candidly about the sadness she has felt as her strength and energy have disappeared from her. Kathy made the observation that she would bet that Mom was probably still running the show from her bed. Mom smiled real big and said, "You can bet on that. I am still the Momma!" I gave her a big high five on hearing her make that statement.

I talked with Kathy about the possibility of increasing Mom's scheduled oxycontin pain medication. I felt she was having to use quite a bit of extra pain medicine to keep her pain under control. Kathy called and got the ok from Doctor B. for the increase.

After Kathy left, Mom was ready for lunch. Earlier in the morning she had asked me to make some more creamy potato salad. She decided that she wanted a big bowl for lunch. It really pleased me to see her really enjoy eating lunch. I had pulled out some *Taste of Home* magazines for her to see if there were any recipes she wanted to cut out and save. She worked on that a while and shortly fell asleep. I felt like I had to wake her up because I thought she had had an accident. As it turns out, it was a false alarm. I explained to Mom that I was trying to be so very careful about keeping her skin clean from any irritants. She told me that she understood and it was better to be safe than sorry.

Mom was pleased when she got a phone call from Bryant. He told Mom that he was on line again and had sent her an email. I printed out the letter for Mom to read and then she put it with all her other notes and cards. Fausto, our volunteer, came by to help with watering Mom's garden. Before he started watering, he came in and visited with Mom for a short while. She enjoys his youth and enthusiasm. Mom had fallen asleep when Fausto was through with the watering. I assured him that I would tell Mom that he enjoyed being in her garden.

I decided to wake Mom, so I could help her with her bath before we ate dinner. Mom chose to sit in the shower chair to take a shower.

Becky or Mom's aides have helped Mom with her bathing. I was a newcomer to this task. I know Mom felt like she had all of the three stooges helping her with a fairly simple task. I had no doubt that I would be able to succeed with helping Mom, because I use a hand-held shower wand when I shower. I think the steam in the bathroom caused my IQ to drop dangerously low. Mom did not even try to hide her shock and displeasure at my unique showering style. Grace was enjoying rolling on the wet bath rug. I told Mom that, at least she didn't have me joining Grace for a roll in her rug. She responded with, "My shower isn't over and it looks like anything is possible with your interpretation of what constitutes a shower." Mom survived the experience and we had our dinner. Mom looked startled and told me that she had to get to the bathroom quickly. Unfortunately, we were not quick enough. She ended up having three more accidents that involved sheets and nightgowns being changed. She became tearful and told me that she did not understand why this was happening to her. She also pointed out, that she had made it through most of the day and was able to eat her oatmeal without any problem. She went on to profusely apologize to me for having to help her with this kind of problem. I told her that if I had to guess, I would think that the combination of radiation enteritis and her tumor causing a sensation of pressure and fullness right at her anus, was having a significant impact on her being able to always have control of her bowels. I asked her to remember how calm and efficient I had been when I have helped her. She admitted that I seemed to be dealing with that task without any signs of discomfort on my part. I told her that I could not say that I was that accomplished with assisting with baths or showers. I told her I felt sad, that I could not protect her from having to endure such indignities, but I was the kind of daughter that was at ease in providing whatever type of personal care she needed, maybe with the exception of showering. She smiled at me and patted my hand.

I got her tucked in and said our prayers for the night. It was a 4-honk night. Fortunately for Mom there were no accidents.

Thank you God, for this day so sweet, for the comfort of a warm bowl of oatmeal, for Mom sharing her feelings about her fatigue and weakness, for the pleasure Mom and I feel when we immerse ourselves in *Taste of Home* magazines, for Mom's sense of humor in dealing with my unique interpretation of showering and for your gift of courage to Mom and me that allowed us to not hide, but to share with each other our feelings and tears about the loss of control Mom is experiencing with her body. Love, Sue

NOVEMBER 4, 2001

Mom had a good day yesterday. We start our days now with shaved ice along with her ice water and cold coke. She really enjoys the shaved ice the most and will ask for it frequently during the day.

Uncle William and Aunt MM stopped by for a short visit. They had found this wonderful fleece-like bed jacket for Mom. Shortly after they left, Becky, Tom and Sherri came in carrying groceries, nightgowns and an electric blanket for her bed. Mom and I both got excited when we heard Grace announce their arrival. It is like we are watching this wondrous magic show pass through our house. Like magic, all the groceries one could want appeared. Like magic, Sherri cleans the patio, feeds the birds, cleans out the somewhat scary front hall closet and hangs out my autumn windsock. Like magic, Tom cleans and repairs the dining room window and also the living room windows, he moves the door jams higher up on the wall, so my oxygen tubing will no longer get caught and cause me to speak in other languages and he makes an adjustment on Mom's basket on her walker that will keep it more stable. Like magic, Becky sweeps through the house dusting, vacuuming, mopping, scrubbing and freshening all that she comes in contact with. If she comes in contact with you, it is in your best interest not to struggle-you will be freshened, so try and enjoy it. Like magic, a beauty parlor is set up and Mom's hair is washed, styled and sprayed into Mom's signature hairstyle. They hug us goodbye and thank us for having a wonderful time. Did you get the part, where they Thank Us! Becky, Tom and Sherri are perfect examples of how a family pulls together to do whatever would be helpful in a time of crisis. All the hard work is really not magic, but it feels that way on the receiving end of all their hard work.

Mom ended up sleeping most of the afternoon. She is taking that extra dose of oxycontin and it will make her sleepy for a few days. Bryant stopped by for a visit. Mom had a chance to catch up on the news about Jacob and Sara and how they are settling into their new home. Bryant could not stay long because he was in the middle of picking up and dropping off these folks that had rented a limo for the night.

Thank you God, for this day so sweet, for the pleasure Mom receives from shaved ice, for the gift of our family's love, which is made not only tangible, but visible to all, for the gift of a peaceful night. Love, Sue

NOVEMBER 5, 2001

Yesterday was filled with some ups and downs for Mom. Our morning started off with a wonderful surprise. Lisa, our next door neighbor, called and said that she was bringing over a breakfast casserole for Mom and me. How wonderful it is to have this kind of surprise happen. After we finished eating, Frances and Babe stopped by for a visit. I enjoy watching the two of them banter back and forth. It is so obvious that they are sisters that love and value each other. I printed out the morning email for Mom to read. She was pleased to find that, in addition to Jenny's note, Bryant had sent her a note. After reading her emails, she continued cutting out recipes from *The Taste of Home* magazines. Uncle William and Aunt MM stopped by after church.

He and Aunt FiFi both have an incredible memory for details. I love hearing them reminisce about their childhood. Mom got real sleepy and napped for most of the day. I feel sure that the increased sedation from her increase in pain medicine will soon subside. I kind of rattled through the house as Mom slept. It dawned on me that when Mom is gone how empty the house will be. Grief work offers many unexpected opportunities to repeatedly deal with painful realities again and again. For the first time, I found myself reading some of the older letters I had written about Mom. I was surprised at how comforted I felt by the words. I was also comforted by the knowledge that my memories may get fuzzy with time, but I will always have my morning letters about Mom.

Later in the afternoon Mom started having episodes with nausea and vomiting. I wonder if the nausea is a result of the increase in her pain medicine. I particularly feel helpless when I am at her bedside and she is pleading to God that he relieve her of her suffering. I do the only thing I can do and that is pray that Mom will feel comforted by God. I had prepared dinner, but Mom was unable to eat. I had given her extra compazine for nausea and it added to her level of sedation.

Diane called to check on Mom. She told me that she might be able to come to see Mom soon. She feels like she is at a point at work where she can take some time off and come be with her Mom. As my older sister, her words of comfort are not only welcomed, but treasured by me. When Mom woke, I told her that Diane had called. She was pleased to hear that her first born would be coming for a visit soon. She also reassured me that she would honk for me if she got hungry or needed anything during the night. She did not honk for me. I can only hope that she didn't need me because she felt that she was stable enough to care for herself.

Thank you God, for this day so sweet, for Uncle William and Aunt FiFi and their shared childhood memories, for the much needed comfort I was blessed with, for compazine and for seeing us safely through the night. Love, Sue

NOVEMBER 6, 2001

Mom had a quiet day yesterday. She complained of not feeling well but there wasn't any one big problem area. She expressed concern that she was going to get nauseated and vomit like she did yesterday evening. She also reminded me that she wasn't going to eat unless she was hungry. I was not given any reasons why. I suspect it does have to do with all the accidents she had, plus her episodes of nausea. What I don't want to consider is that she might be passively trying to decrease the amount of time she has left with us. I know she is so very weary and eating is a big struggle for her. Maybe she is not wanting to struggle anymore. If the opportunity presents itself, I intend to talk to her about her feelings, about the problems she has in trying to eat. I did decide to gently encourage her to try and eat, but not push. I would strongly encourage that she keep up her fluid intake. Becoming dehydrated impacts how her medicines are absorbed.

I could tell that my anxiety level went up because I spent the entire day in the kitchen cooking. As a psychiatric nurse, I would consider this peculiar behavior and worth an hour on the couch, processing my feelings. Before Mom talked to me about her decision, I had planned on doing some cooking today, but not spend the whole day cooking. I made a meatloaf with a glaze, frozen fruit salad, Aunt Lois's yeast roll dough, baked egg custard, navy bean soup with ham and new potatoes to go with the meatloaf. Mom did eat maybe eight ounces of the broth from the navy bean soup. When I told her that the egg custard was wonderful she asked for a cup of custard, which she promptly polished off. I was so happy that I went and prepared an extra batch, in case she would want extra custard.

In the middle of my cooking marathon, Mom and I had a wonderful surprise, Diane's package with gifts for Mom arrived. When I opened it up, I got distracted by the enormous quantity of bubble wrap. I immediately commenced to popping bubbles. Mom was able to finally get my attention and asked if that was the surprise Diane had sent her. I put the bubble wrap down and found Mom's surprise from Diane. It was a clear acrylic pocket that fits on the side rail of her hospital bed. It will be real handy for things like the phone, remote control, magazines and other small things. Mom was so excited that she wanted me to call Diane right then. I had to leave a message, but she quickly returned our call. I told Diane that there were other things in the box, like two tins of Bert's Lip Balm, two large print *Reader's Digest* magazines, two books on *How to Revive Your Brain* and a plastic foot shaped brush you put it in the tub or shower and you can scrub the bottom of your feet without losing balance. Diane told me that there had been a mistake in the order. She had not ordered any of Bert's balm or the *Reader's Digest* or *How to Revive Your Brain*. She did order the foot scrubber for me as a surprise. The surprise foot scrubber in combination with the bubble wrap sent me right over the edge. Mom started arranging her personal stuff in her new pockets. We both were having a wonderful early Christmas. It would have been perfect if Diane could have been here to hear us chatting, laughing about the *Revive Your Brain* books and popping bubbles all at the same time. There is a lot to be said for how unexpected surprises can really brighten one's day.

I printed out Mom's email and she enjoyed her notes from Jenny and Bryant. After reading her mail, she decided to take a short nap. Gracie's barking at the mailman woke Mom from her nap. There were Christmas catalogs and her daily note from her sister. Mom and I thumbed through the catalogs and found perfect Christmas presents for everyone. The only problem was that you would have had to win the lottery to be able to pay for all of it. It is a lot of fun to look at the pictures and get swept away with all the magic on the pages. It is a stress reliever for me.

Mom surprised me by eating all of her dinner. I had put very small portions on her plate. When I say small, I mean maybe two or three bites worth of food. After *The Antique Roadshow* was over Mom and I said our prayers and I tucked her in tight for the night. Mom did not honk for me last night. She is still sleeping and looks ok.

Thank you God, for this day so sweet, for Diane who sends wonderful surprises that take you to a happy and carefree place, for comfort foods like egg custard and for that big box of bubble wrap with enough bubbles to handle any future stress or strain. Love, Sue

Baked Custard

2 eggs
2 Tbs sugar
½ tsp nutmeg
1/4 tsp salt
2 cups milk scalded
   Beat eggs
   Add sugar, nutmeg and salt
   Gradually stir in the scalded milk into the egg mixture
   Pour mixture into custard cups
   Place custard cups on a cake pan on the oven rack
   Pour hot water till it almost reaches the top of the cups
   Bake at 325° for about 30 minutes or until knife blade comes out clean
   Don't cook too long

NOVEMBER 7, 2001

Yesterday was full of visitors and feelings of helplessness. Mom wanted oatmeal for breakfast and I was excited at the prospect of Mom eating. She was only able to eat a few bites. Mom told me that it felt like she was choking on it. I offered to prepare something else and she told me maybe later she would eat something. Vicky, Mom's aide, arrived early. Mom and I both were happy to see her. I know Mom wasn't looking forward to having another "near bath" experience with me. After Vicky left, Mom started having accidents. She could not seem to get to the bathroom in time. You could tell how absolutely worn out she was after having to get cleaned up five times. I finally gave her an Immodium in hopes of slowing her gut down. She assured me that she would be ok with Marilyn staying with her for a short time, while I ran a couple of errands. Mom's tummy had calmed down and I decided to go on and get out after Marilyn arrived.

I picked up some salt risen bread for Mom and then went to the Sample House. They had all their Christmas decorations out. I spent some time just looking and was surprised to find myself near tears. I left the store and went and sat in the car for a while. I found myself thinking about whether Mom would even be here for Christmas and if she was here, what kind of condition she would be in. I pulled myself together and went to the store to pick up some dishwashing liquid and a *National Enquirer* for Mom. She and I both secretly find tabloid news entertaining. It is embarrassing to buy it, but I do it for Mom.

Before I had left the house, I had heated up a small cup of the broth from the Navy Bean soup for Mom. Her almost full cup of soup was one of the first things I noticed when I returned from my outing. She caught my eye and quietly told me that she was doing the best that she could. I patted her hand and told her that I knew she was doing her very best. Mom told me that Kathy had just left and was going to check with Dr. B. about some Raglan. She felt like it might help with Mom's swallowing. Marilyn and Mom seemed to have enjoyed themselves while I was gone. Maryanne, the social worker, arrived as Marilyn was leaving. She spent some time talking to Mom, and then Mom got tired and wanted to cut short her visit. Marianne asked me if I wanted to talk for a while. Again, I found myself totally swept away with tears. Marianne talked about how hard it was to find that your nurturing was not making it all better. To feed someone you love is such an important and very basic way we show our love. I know Mom is struggling with the whole idea of eating. I am also struggling with the idea that no matter what I prepare, Mom is eating less and less. Marianne talked about her mother's final days and her food cravings. Marianne would prepare her mother's comfort foods and her mother was only able to take a few bites before she would feel full. That is what Mom is doing right now. Marianne told me that it was also painful for her to watch her mother eat less and less each day. Painful is one of the words to describe the feelings that surround this front row seat I occupy. I also expressed fear that I might be developing pleurisy. This is the first time that I have even thought about what would happen if I got sick. I did a lot of crying about that before I was able to look at my back-up plans in caring for Mom. Marianne reminded me that they did offer respite care, but she had a feeling that my family and friends would pull together to make sure Mom was taken care of. I know that Mom and I can count on having all the support that we could need. I told Maryanne that if I did not feel better in the morning I would call my doctor. The good news is that it is morning and I am not having chest pains anymore. After Marianne left, I went to check on Mom and found her sleeping. The phone rang and it was Becky checking in on us. The minute I heard her voice I started to cry. Becky wanted to come right over. I told her it wasn't necessary. I was in a place where what I needed most to do was to cry. She offered to come spend the night. Again, I told her that caring for Mom was, for the most part, emotionally draining. It was just a comfort to talk to her on the phone. I told her that we would all go through this part of grieving. This just happened to be my turn. She told me that the box that had been delivered was for me. I was surprised when I opened it and found my favorite signature fragrance. Clinique's "Aromatics." Becky's timing is right on the money. I had a few sprays of perfume left before I would have been out.

When Mom woke, I told her that my eyes were red because I was not feeling well and I was also feeling sad that I was unable to make things easier for her. She patted my hand and made me promise to call the doctor in the morning. She also told me that I really was making a lot of things easier for her to deal with. She told me to get the Bengay cream and she would rub my back. Before I went to get the cream, I offered an egg custard to her and she accidentally spilled it. I told her not to worry, that I could have some hot egg custard ready for her in about forty minutes. While the custard was cooking, Mom did finish a small cup of navy bean soup. She surprised me when she was able to eat all of her custard. I was aware of the wheels spinning in my head about how I could fix all sort of custards, puddings and gelatin desserts. I was also acutely aware that the wheels spinning in my head were actually a reflection of my heart's struggle with the ever growing reality of having to say goodbye to my mother.

I went to call Diane to talk with her about all of this and Mom started honking for me. We were having a repeat of this morning's activities. I was having mixed feelings of sadness and anger that Mom was so weak and having to struggle with the loss of a basic bodily function. After the fourth trip to the bathroom, I gave her another immodium. I tucked her in and we said our prayers. I said an extra prayer that Mom would be able to completely rest after such an exhausting day. I called Diane back and we both shared some tears together. She reminded me that it won't be too much longer before she will be coming for a visit.

I am really looking forward to seeing her. We both decided to try and escape into the season premier of NYPD Blue. Before the show started, I called Lynda and asked her if she could come over in the morning and help me hook up Mom's VCR. I had a movie from Blockbuster that I thought she would enjoy. I was crying before I was able to ask her for help with the VCR. She reassured me that she will come first thing in the morning. I pulled myself together and climbed into bed to watch *NYPD Blue.*

Mom honked 1 time during the night.

It was 44° this morning. The cats were impressed with my moon-walk.

Thank you God, for this day so sweet, for the time Marianne spent with me, for Becky's thoughtfulness, for my Mom's back rub, for egg custard warm from the oven, for shared tears with Diane, for Lynda being there when I needed her, for a 44° morning and for the awareness that I felt physically well and my chest pain was gone. Love, Sue

NOVEMBER 8, 2001

Yesterday was a good day for Mom. The day started off with a soft feel to it. Mom slept late and when she woke, she was smiling and asking for her morning toast. I sat on the end of her bed and we told each other what we dreamed about. Lynda arrived with milk and eggs. I am using quite a bit in making the baked egg custards for Mom. Lynda had a picture of her great grandson, Andrew, dressed as a frog for Halloween. Mom and I just melted when we saw this big green frog named Andrew. Before we knew it, Mom had fallen asleep.

When Lynda and I had some time alone the tears started again. I told her that earlier, when I was typing out my morning note, that I did not know if I was going to be able to finish the note because of the quantity of tears I was producing. I told her that it was important to me that I complete my morning notes. I suggested that we watch a movie because I could use some major distraction. My eyes were almost swollen shut from all the crying. We tried watching this drama, but it was lost on us. We decided that "Songcatcher" might do the trick. It was about a musicologist attempting to record early 20th century ballads in the Appalachian Mountains. It was just what the doctor ordered. Mom slept soundly while we watched the movie. Bryant came by to check on Mom, but she never woke up. Marianne called to check on me. She was relieved to hear that the chest pain I was experiencing had gone and also that I had called Lynda to spend some time with me.

A neighbor stopped by to visit with Mom. Fortunately Mom woke up and was able to visit with her. Shortly after she left, Mom was asleep again. Lynda needed to scoot home. We made plans for tomorrow for her to come and stay with Mom while I got out. Mom woke shortly before dinner and wanted to get up and walk around. We ended up in the kitchen and she showed me her secret for blender slaw. She mentioned that she would like to get something that would fit in the acrylic pocket on her bedside rail to help organize her pens, index cards, stamps and paper clips. When I mentioned the Container Store she told me she was ready to go. I told her that she had a deal. We would plan on going tomorrow after my oxygen had been delivered. She sat at the table and ate most of her dinner.

After watching *The Appraisal Fair,* we said our prayers and turned in for the night. It was a 1-honk night.

When I let Grace out, I noticed that the temperature was a disappointing 52°. At least they say we will be having a cold front moving in today.

Thank you God, for this day so sweet, for a frog named Andrew, for the company of a good friend, for Mom showing me her secret to wonderful slaw, for a shared dinner in the kitchen and for the excitement of making plans with Mom to go shopping. Love, Sue

Secret Blender Slaw

SALAD INGREDIENTS

1 large head of cabbage

1 Large bell pepper

1 large onion

DRESSING

1 cup vinegar

3/4 cup sugar

1 ½ tsp salt

1 tsp celery seed

3/4 cup oil

Hunk cabbage, onion and peppers and put into blender

Repeat until all is shredded

Of course, you can do it by hand if you want to

Cover with water and shred for about 2 seconds (Watch it or you can really mess it up)

Pour into colander to drain

Boil first four dressing ingredients for 2 minutes

Remove from heat and add oil

Bring to boil again and pour over cabbage

Cover tightly, place in refrigerator and let it remain overnight

Makes 2 quarts

NOVEMBER 9, 2001

Mom had a nice day yesterday. First thing we talked about that morning was our plans to go shopping. We both were so excited at the thought of getting out. Mom had not been grocery shopping since August. Mom got up and chose the clothes she was going to wear on her outing. We were surprised to find that Lynda and Andrew had come for a visit. Andrew held onto Lynda's fingers and walked across the room. He is growing up so fast. Lynda said that they came to join in on our pre-celebration activities. She surprised us with thoughtful gifts for Mom, Gracie and me. Mom was excited to find that she now has her very own salsa bowl, decorated with peppers. I was excited over a birdseed that was bell-shaped. Gracie is really styling with a bandana with diamonds on it. (We can call them diamonds if we want to). Andrew showed us all the new things he has learned to do. Mom and I really enjoyed the unexpected opportunity to visit with Andrew and Lynda.

Mom decided to take a short nap before lunch. I piddled around and made Mom some baked egg custard. Mom woke up and ate her lunch. We started counting down the time till we would leave on our shopping adventure. We waited and waited for my oxygen to be delivered. I finally wrote a note and put it on the front door for John, my oxygen delivery guy. Mom, Lynda and I loaded up and took off. We were a couple of blocks away from our house and Mom had a short episode of dry heaves. She wanted to continue with our shopping experience. They stopped after a few minutes. I wish I knew what was causing her to have problems with episodes of dry heaves.

We first went to Kroger to pick up the ingredients for a special recipe she wanted to prepare. We then headed out to the Container Store. It was exciting to find all their Christmas wrapping paper and ribbons on display. We found some small bags and containers that will hold the assortment of things that Mom wants to keep at her bedside. She was so tired when we got home that she did not take off her slacks before she laid down. Before dinner I helped her get her nightgown on.

Diane called to check on Mom. I am so excited to think about the possibility of her coming next weekend. Mom said she would like to get out again. She was quick to say that did not mean the next day, but soon.

We both turned in early for the night. Mom did not honk for me during the night.

Thank you God, for this day so sweet, for the gift of being able to get Mom out of her bed, out of the house and a chance to go shopping and for Diane's phone call that held the promise of her coming for a visit. Love, Sue

NOVEMBER 10, 2001
Jenny is Diane's daughter. Gordon is Diane's husband who is very ill.

Yesterday was a nice day for Mom. She got up and had her toast at the kitchen table. Instead of going back to bed, she sat in the recliner and looked at Christmas catalogs. Kathy soon arrived for her assessment on Mom's health status. There were no changes in Mom's medications. Mom decided to take a nap before lunch. It was a gray, overcast day and was conducive for nap taking.

I don't usually take naps during the day, but I laid down for a while. When we got up, Mom wanted to make a No Peek Stew. She sat at the table and told me step by step what went into the stew. I can't begin to describe how good it felt to have her in the kitchen with me. We had finished up in the kitchen and it was time for Mom's afternoon soap opera. I printed out her emails. She was pleased to, not only get her daily note from Jenny, but she got a note from Carol and Margie.

Mom surprised me by wanting to have dinner at the kitchen table. I am focusing on the joy of the moment because that is all any of us have. Diane called after dinner and talked with Mom. We both were so happy to hear that Diane might come at the end of next week and spend Thanksgiving with us. I want to take the opportunity right now to thank Jenny and Billy for staying home to take care of Gordon and the animals. I know that Jenny is most eager to be with her Granny. She also realizes how precious it will be for her Mom to have a chance to spend some time alone with her mother. The gift of time with Mom is the most precious gift one could receive at this point. When she talked with me, I was so excited when she told me that she had a new computer for me. I have been having to nurse mine along and hope that it will make it for my morning notes about Mom. Mom just smiled as Diane and I were giggling over the excitement of my new computer.

Becky called to make sure we had a nice afternoon and to tell us that she would be coming by herself tomorrow. Mom and I spent some time talking about what she wanted to do for Christmas for Becky and Tom.

It was soon time for our bedtime prayers. Mom did not honk during the night.

Thank you God, for this day so sweet, for the gift of Mom's guidance as I put together the stew, for the emails that brightened her day, for Diane's call that left Mom and me with big grins on our faces and in our hearts and for Jenny's precious gift of time that will allow Mom and Diane to be together at Thanksgiving. Love, Sue

No Peek Stew

2 pounds stew meat
1 cup potatoes
1 cup sliced celery
1 cup onion quartered
1 cup sliced carrots
2 tbs tapioca
2 cans Snap-E-Tom
Salt, pepper, Season All
    Dissolve tapioca in Snap-E-Tom—pour over meat and vegetables
    Cover and bake 5 hours at 250°

NOVEMBER 11, 2001

Mom had a very nice day yesterday. First thing she did in the morning was to walk around the house and check on the front and back yard. She then decided to have her morning toast at the kitchen table. Becky soon arrived with groceries in hand. She helped Mom with her bath. Mom and I were both relieved that I was not involved. Becky worked her magic in the house and soon it was time for her to head home.

Mom and I both had a quiet afternoon. After dinner we watched some TV, then turned in for the night. It was a 1-honk night.

Thank you God, for this day so sweet, for our Saturdays with Becky and for the peaceful comfort of a day of shared quiet times. Love, Sue

NOVEMBER 12, 2001

Yesterday was a very sleepy day for Mom. Unfortunately, I have to keep this note very short because this is the third time I have tried to complete it. I would almost be through and the computer freezes on me. Hopefully, I can do some maintenance and get out a regular note tomorrow. Love, Sue

NOVEMBER 13, 2001

The last several days Mom has been very sleepy and has had zero appetite. Mom did wake up on Sunday with a very swollen right hand and right foot. I wondered about her kidneys, but it would not be happening on just one side. I decided to call Kathy on Monday and ask her about having some blood work done on Mom. Hospice doesn't pay for blood work, so it would be out of pocket. On Sunday Mom had a fried egg in a hole and one small taquito. Monday morning I coaxed her to eat one piece of toast. She fell asleep right after eating her toast.

When I gave her the morning pain pills, I was surprised when she refused them. She had decided that maybe she was allergic to them.

125

Nothing I said would convince her otherwise. She wanted to talk to Kathy and see what she had to say. I called Kathy and she told Mom what I had told her and she proceeded to take her medication. I was pleased to see that she had developed such a trusting relationship with Kathy. I am still surprised that she would not accept my explanations.

After she took her medicine, she was asleep again. I finally woke her at 12:30 and told her she needed to wake up and drink some water and try to eat something. She flatly said that the only thing she was interested in was some cold water. I knew it would probably make her mad, but I woke her up at 3:30 and told her that if she did not eat something, she would be too weak to walk to the bathroom. She did say she would try some of the broth from the navy bean soup. She probably consumed maybe six ounces. She has been doing marathon sleeping, like she had done some weeks ago. On top of all the sleeping, she is not eating. A neighbor had brought over some chicken and dumplings. Mom told me that she would try to eat some for dinner. She ate maybe half of a cup. She was able to stay awake and watch part of *The Antique Roadshow*. It was hard dealing with Mom sleeping 20 out of 24 hours several weeks ago. To have to deal with her not eating on top of sleeping all the time is doubly hard. I don't think that she has consumed more that 500 calories in the last two days. My role as her primary care giver involves making sure she takes her pain pills and her laxatives each day. I can put out her other medication, but I am not supposed to pressure her. She knows what pills she needs to take and if she chooses not to, so be it. I can gently encourage her to drink, but if she refuses to eat, I am supposed to back off. I also make sure that she stays clean, dry and comfortable. It is so hard not to make a frenzied effort to make things right with Mom again. I have my hands tied as I watch her pull further and further away from me. No matter how hard it is for me, I will not harass Mom about her eating, sleeping or what medicine she takes. I am thankful that I cannot only tell her I love her, but show her by respecting her wishes.

Mom did not honk for me last night.

Thank you God, for this day so sweet, for homemade chicken and dumplings and for the gift of courage to nurture Mom in ways that are comforting to her at this point in her journey. Love, Sue

NOVEMBER 14, 2001

Mom had a nice day yesterday. Kathy came first thing in the morning to check on Mom. She was also perplexed about the localized swelling in her right hand and right foot. She said she would talk to Dr. B. about her symptoms. Mom also expressed concern about how sleepy she was. In fact, during the assessment, Mom complained of having difficulty in staying awake. I suddenly found myself tearing up while Kathy and I talked about Mom's lack of food intake. Mom did not see my tears, but she did hear me speak of wanting to provide for her and how I understood in my head that she will eat when she feels like she can.

Mom did take a nap after Kathy left. I focused on trying to get my computer to send my morning message out. It kept freezing up on me. I was surprised to later find that it went out around 2 p.m. If you don't get a morning note from me in the next couple of days, just know it is because I am having trouble with it.

The good news is that Diane is bringing a brand-new one to me this week end. It is so powerful that I don't even have to worry about cleaning out the cat box or loading the dishwasher-it does it for me! It will be a most wonderful early Christmas present. Diane laughed a long time ago, when I asked her if my computer had Advance Directives. She is not laughing now, with all the peculiar things it is doing as it is in its final days. Lynda came over around 1:30 to stay with Mom while I went to search for the perfect pre-lit Christmas tree. A replacement aide named Paige came to assist Mom with her bath. Lynda and I noticed that Mom had a scary look on her face as she interacted with Paige. After an intense conversation it was decided that she could change her bed and then leave. Paige was a rather tall very muscular woman that had a "no nonsense" attitude about her. If I was in Mom's shoes, I would have been alarmed at the idea of how hard she might scrub my back. Lynda told me to go on and begin my mission and she and Mom would work everything out. I did find the perfect tree for the living room and also a small three foot tree with 100 multicolor lights on it for Mom's room. I am going to put Mom's tree on her tall chest at the foot of her bed. When I realized that I was going to have to somehow get this very heavy box into the trunk I started to say a prayer. My problems were solved when the checker turned off her register light and found a young man that was able to get the box in the trunk, tie it down and had a big happy smile on his face when he was through. It is so refreshing to stumble upon people that provide service with a smile.

When I got home, I discovered wonderful smells from the kitchen and Lynda humming a song. Mom had just laid down for a nap. Lynda told me that she and Mom had a very nice day. Mom allowed her to help her with her personal care. After she got cleaned up, she asked Lynda for a cup of soup which she promptly consumed. They then spent some time looking at Christmas catalogs. Mom also got up and walked around the house checking on things. Lynda told me that they had a wonderful afternoon.

My day could not have been better. Mom was awake, eating and chatting with Lynda, not to mention that I had found two perfect trees. Lynda was making chicken fried steak fingers, gravy, mashed potatoes and peas. I struggled to find the words to thank her for the gift of this day. She is always available to help out at any time, but she will appear at times when Mom and I both need a major break from each other. I had not been looking forward to spending another day watching Mom not eat. I was so pleased that she did develop a little appetite while I was gone. Mom cleaned her plate at dinner and even wanted seconds on the mashed potatoes and gravy.

After Lynda left, Mom and I got ready for the night. We both had many things to give thanks for in our evening prayers. I was sitting at the computer at 9 p.m. when I heard the most horrible screaming come from Mom's room. Grace and I thundered down the hall, not knowing what we would find. I had to give Mom several hard shakes to wake her up. When she opened her eyes, she grabbed me and said, "I knew that you would come and rescue me." She told me that she had been dreaming that this man was stabbing her. Mom had another dream like this one a couple of years back. A doctor I was working with called the dreams hypnogogic dreams. They are the worst kind of nightmare dreams.

All I know is that after Mom went back to sleep. Grace and I were both so rattled that we took a nerve pill and snuggled together.

It was a 2-honk night.

Thank you God, for this day so sweet, for the sweet comfort of Lynda's friendship, for the much needed help in the Wal-Mart parking lot and for second helpings of mashed potatoes and gravy. Love, Sue

NOVEMBER 15, 2001

Mom had a quiet day yesterday. She spent a good majority of the time sleeping. She came to the kitchen table and ate her morning toast. We talked about her nightmare. I told her that when I heard her piercing scream. I was sure that something had snapped off. The basic fear for me was that the mass had perhaps eroded through the bladder or rectal wall. Her colorectal doctor expressed concern that there was an up and down side to not having liver metastasis. The down side was that it gave the tumor plenty of time to erode through anything it could reach. I have no idea what would happen if it would erode through the wall of her bladder. He is the one that also said that Mom would likely get weaker and weaker and just fade away. That certainly seems to be happening.

Moving on. She sat at the table and marked things in catalogs that she would like to order for friends and family. While she was sitting at the table, she gave me directions on how to prepare Mildred's vegetable salad. She wanted to be sure that Marilyn had the salad while her brother was visiting her. It was a moment that I have savored and put in a special place for the future.

Bryant came by for a short visit and was pleased to find Mom sitting at the kitchen table. He was not able to stay long because he had a doctor's appointment. Not long after Bryant left, Mom started with dry heaves. It lasted for about five minutes then it was gone. I still don't understand that symptom. I helped her back to bed and she slept till I woke her for lunch. I gave her a selection of small finger food appetizers. She did eat one of the appetizers. I told her to let me know if she wanted to have soup or anything else later in the day. I was pleased to see her eat some shaved ice. At 2 p.m. she had another dry heave episode and I decided to try an Ativan, to help ease the symptoms. She told me about half an hour later that she felt very relaxed and calm. It also made her sleepy and she slept for the rest of the afternoon. I spent some time printing her emails from Margie and Jenny for her to read later. I never know when my computer will cooperate and not cop an attitude with me. I have two more days and then I will have brand new wheels, so to speak.

Mom was very sleepy when I woke her for dinner. She had trouble keeping her eyes open long enough to eat. She did eat two bites of her meatloaf, mashed potatoes and green beans. Diane and I talked about her planned arrival on this coming Saturday. It will be so absolutely wonderful to have her here 24 hours a day for a week. Not to mention, all of us being able to spend time with Mom. After we had said our prayers, I leaned down to kiss Mom on her forehead. I told her I loved her the most and she sleepily responded, "There is no way anyone could love you as much as I do." I became tearful. She told me that they better be tears of happiness. I assured her they were happy tears. Many people will go through life doubting that they were ever loved. I have never doubted it, but being reminded of that love right before bedtime was special.

Mom did not honk last night.

Thank you God, for this day so sweet, for unexpected memory making time in the kitchen with Mom, for the joy Mom and I feel when we think about Saturday and for the cherished knowledge that my Mother loves me totally and completely. Love, Sue

NOVEMBER 16, 2001

Yesterday was a very sleepy day for Mom. I had to wake her up at 8:30, so she could take her pain medicine and go to the bathroom. Vicky, Mom's aide, arrived shortly after Mom got back in bed. Mom and I both were very happy to see that she felt well enough to work today. Mom feels very comfortable with Vicky's way of assisting her with her bath and the way she makes her bed. We were both excited to find out that starting this coming Monday she will be returning to her regular Monday, Wednesday and Friday schedule with Mom. Mom was only able to eat half a piece of toast. I used to toast two pieces of bread for her, but for the last two weeks I have toasted only one piece. I don't think that it will ever get any easier to watch her eat less and less. It is such a huge reminder that she cannot survive very long on a very small number of calories. The thought of her maybe not being here for Christmas has been weighing heavy on my mind. She has no reserve to fall back on. I am now able to see how she loses a little more ground each day. This is the first time that I have allowed myself to

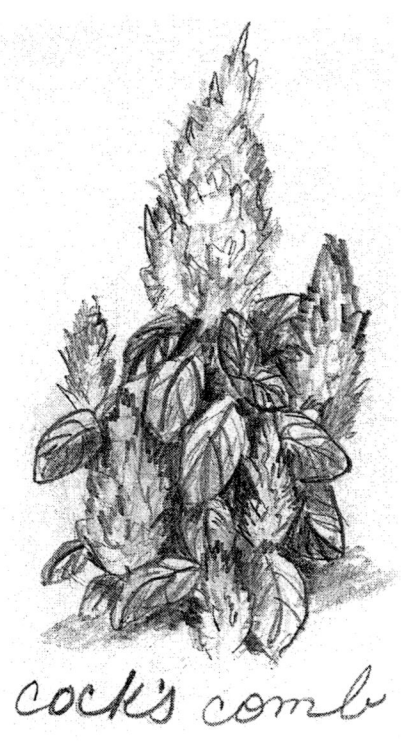

cock's comb

acknowledge out loud, that the pace of her physical decline has accelerated. I often wonder if there is something I have not said or done that I should be doing while she is alert and aware. I don't feel like I could begin to tell her enough times how thankful I am to have been blessed with such a remarkable Mother and how deeply I love her. In my head, I know that she has heard those words and believes me when I have told her my feelings. I think that there are probably never enough words or time to tell our mothers how much they are loved and how much they will be missed when they are gone.

Lynda came over after Vicky had left. Mom had fallen asleep shortly after Vicky had left. Lynda and I had some time to talk about our mothers. Lynda's mother died about 3 years ago. She tells me that at times, it feels just like it happened yesterday. She went on to say that there are times that it does get easier. We both shed some tears together. Both of us have enjoyed wonderful relationships with our mothers as adults.

Mom finally woke at 1:30 and asked for a cup of soup. She drank maybe six ounces. I was thankful for those six ounces. It wasn't very long before she was asleep again. I spent some time going through my email and printing the notes from Jenny and Margie for Mom. Margie wrote such a wonderful note, reminiscing about the times they shared in high school. She also had some very kind words of encouragement for me. It was unexpected, but much appreciated.

Mom woke around 5 p.m. She was trying to orient herself. It was dark in her room because it was raining. She sat up in bed and we looked at catalogs together. Both of us were taking turns having each other to take a peek at something wonderful that we had just discovered. Needless to say, it was a sweet time.

She was able to eat about a half a cup of Shepherds pie and a piece of toast. Soon after dinner, she was asleep again and did not wake until 5 the next morning.

Thank you God, for this day so sweet, for Vicky's tender touch with Mom, for the time with Lynda and for the gift of time after dinner with Mom. Love, Sue

NOVEMBER 17, 2001

Yesterday was another very sleepy day for Mom. She woke up as I finished writing my morning note. Mom noticed that I had some tears in my eyes. I viewed this as opportunity for me to tell Mom what was weighing heavily in my heart. I told her that the tears were mostly tears of gratitude, with some sadness mixed in. I began to tell her about what I had just written in my morning note. I told her that I was happy to have this moment to share what I was feeling. I continued to talk about how I knew that I was always loved, even when, as a youngster, I wasn't behaving in a loving way. I also knew how truly blessed I was, not to mention my sisters and brother, to have a loving, joyful, adult relationship with my mother. She would always be first my mother, but I considered her my best friend. I knew not everybody could say that about their relationship with their mother. I went on to express the fear I have of not being able to find enough ways or words to describe how I loved her and how truly blessed I was to have had her beside me as I grew physically, emotionally and spiritually. I didn't want her to have any doubts about my deep gratitude, for being blessed with such a mother and best friend. She reached over and patted my hand, gave me a hug and told me that she not only knew how I felt, but experienced my love in how I was caring for her now. She wanted me to know that she loved me and felt blessed to have a daughter named Sue. I asked her if she had ever worried that she had left anything unsaid with her mother. Mom told me that she felt like she had said what she needed to say to her mother, but regretted her immaturity when her father was dying. She was a teenager at the time and did not share all that was in her heart with him before he died. It felt so good to be able to sit by Mom and share my tears, fears and love with her.

Mom decided that she was hungry for a piece of toast. We hugged each other and I got up and made her morning toast. She dozed off, soon after eating most of her toast. Janet, the chaplain, came by for a visit. She was only able to have a short visit with Mom because Mom was nauseated and somewhat groggy. Janet and I talked for a while in the kitchen. I felt so supported as we talked. I told her about my morning conversation with Mom. She said that she would come back while Diane was here.

When I checked on Mom, she asked for a fried egg and tomato sandwich. I jumped on that opportunity quickly. I was pleased to see her eat a whole half of a sandwich. After eating, she was soon asleep. Uncle William, Aunt MM and Lee stopped by for a brief visit with Mom. MM brought one of her warm bed jackets for Mom to wear. All of us were talking about how excited we all were to have an opportunity to see Steve and Aunt FiFi, on the Friday after Thanksgiving. He is flying in from Detroit on Thanksgiving Day and will then drive from Denton to Dallas on Friday. I know that this Thanksgiving will be one that we are all acutely aware of our many blessings. Fausto, Mom's volunteer from hospice, came to water the garden and feed the birds. He is taking piano in college and I had encouraged him to bring his piano book so he could practice. It was nice hearing him play the piano. Mom slept till Kathy arrived for her assessment. She had trouble staying awake while Kathy was here. Soon after Kathy and Fausto left, my friend Delbert came by with a pot of hot stew for our dinner.

Mom woke around 5:30 and wanted a bowl of oatmeal. I told her that we had stew. She had gotten her days and nights mixed up. She decided that she still wanted some oatmeal. She took two bites and complained of it hanging in her throat. I asked her if she would try to eat some baked egg custard. She ate maybe five ounces and was asleep.

It was a 6-honk night. Mom complained of feeling restless and thirsty.

Thank you God, for this day so sweet, for the chance to share what was in my heart with Mom, for warm bed jackets and for a friend's homemade stew. Love, Sue

NOVEMBER 18, 2001

Yesterday was a hard day for Mom. She was lethargic and disoriented. I feel like she has become toxic on her pain medicine. Mom has not required any extra pain medicine for days now. The goal of good pain management is no breakthrough pain, but Mom doesn't seem to be metabolizing her pain medicine like she has in the past. I am going to hold her long-acting pain medicine and see if she will clear mentally. I have the short acting to use as a back up if she begins to hurt. I won't let her hurt no matter what.

Becky came early Saturday morning to freshen up the house and bring our groceries. She suggested that we go on and put up the tree, so that it would give the branches a chance to settle. We have never put a tree up before Thanksgiving, but things have been different in our house, and Mom and I could use a little early Christmas cheer. The tree is absolutely perfect. Mom did walk into the living room to take a look at it.

While Becky was here, I took the opportunity to get out and run a few errands. It is so stressful seeing Mom like this. She is aware enough that it bothers her and she complains of feeling crazy. By the time I got back home Mom was sleeping peacefully. Becky and I visited for a while before she had to leave for her home. Mom slept through the afternoon as I waited for Diane's arrival.

This afternoon I found out that our neighbor Sue's father had died. Mom and I have been so close to Sue that this is sad news. Her mom had died two years ago this November and her father had been angry and aloof since that time. She won't have the opportunity for closure, since he died so unexpectedly. She has not seen Mom since early summer. She has apologized for not visiting, but says that she can't begin to face what is happening to Mom. I hope that she will be able to pull herself together before it is too late to say goodbye to Mom.

Diane arrived around 7 p.m. and excitedly came into the house carrying my new computer. Grace got in between her legs and Diane started to fall. Somehow she banked off of the piano bench and rolled, while she held the computer up. It was like thinking that my transplant surgeon was about to drop my new heart on the carpet and then my heart would be ruined because it got covered in dog and cat hair. But she was able at the last moment to save the day, not to mention my heart.

Fortunately, Diane only scraped her knee and the computer survived the incident. In fact, I am already using it. I don't have to live in fear that my computer will freeze up on me. It was hard to watch Diane's face as she saw Mom walk into the kitchen, very slowly and holding tightly to her walker. (I know that it was a painful shock to her system). Diane told Mom that she had a big surprise for her and went to her car to retrieve it. She appeared at the kitchen table holding a beautiful wall-mounted recirculating fountain for Mom's patio wall. I couldn't help myself, I had to call Becky and tell her that the fountain was for her bedroom wall. I have seen fountains like that in magazines. There was total silence on Becky's end of the line. I have never heard her be speechless. I finally broke her silence with the truth. All she could utter was "Yeah, Yeah, Yeah." It sounded almost like a growl. Diane soon snapped out of the shock to her system and began to take inventory of what needed to be done. Those kinds of reflexes run deep. It will be so nice when we call all be together.

I was surprised when Mom told me that she wanted a potato and a tomato for dinner. I added a little roast, roast gravy and three slices of tomatoes. I was further surprised to see her clean her plate. I tried to explain, in simple terms, that I was going to hold her pain medicine at bedtime. She said that she was relieved.

Diane, Mom and I said our prayers together and we kissed her goodnight. Diane immediately sat down and started to remove the cables from my old computer and hook up my new computer. The computer was originally styled to be a "Barbie" computer. The "Barbie" decals have been sanded off, so there are some dull splotches on it. I think it just adds to the aura surrounding this little bubble-shaped computer. It has a silver case with purple buttons and a pink handle on top. It is shaped like those old portable hair dryers we used to have. It even has little silver fins coming out of the back of its case. I showed Diane a catalog that had the perfect accessory for a computer with this kind of fashion statement. I had found these pink, plastic Cadillac fins with adhesive backs on them, so you could mount them on the sides of your computer. I believe in getting into the spirit of things. I was beside myself. I had one talented sister, with stunt women abilities, hook up my new "Burbie" computer. We have to call it "Burbie" because "Barbie" was sanded off.

I did not last as long as Diane did. She is a real night owl. Mom slept till about 4:45 a.m. She honked for help so she could go to the bathroom. She seemed a little clearer to me. Her speech was a lot easier to understand. She remembered that Diane had arrived last evening.

Around 6:30, she was ready for some toast. I decided to wake Diane so she could share morning toast with her Mom. Diane hopped right up and joined Mom at the table. It was wonderful to hear Mom think and speak so clearly. She asked questions about what was going on with our neighbors.

She, later in the morning, laughed at a funny incident that had happened in the bathroom. I was trying to show Diane how I do the ritual morning enema. Mother was going along with the instructions and was faithfully following each one. Diane was standing at the door to the bathroom watching me. I was standing with my back to Mom, so I could provide her with some privacy. I quickly discovered that I had left out the critical part of the instructions regarding nozzle placement prior to releasing the clamp holding the water back. I asked Mom if she was ready for me to hold the bag up and she responded with a big affirmative "yes." When I held the bag up, I suddenly found myself in a torrential downpour. Mom was holding the nozzle up and away from her and I was getting an unintended water treatment. It had Diane laughing so hard she was doubled up. I was trying to regain my composure. Mom told me it was a good lesson on the importance of giving accurate instructions. I am still chuckling about it. It was good to see Mom see the humor in all of it.

Thank you God, for this day so sweet, for multi-talented sisters, for my wondrous new computer and beautiful Christmas tree, for a peaceful night's sleep and for the healing power of humor. Love, Sue

NOVEMBER 20, 2001

Mom had a wonderful day yesterday. We all enjoyed a breakfast of scrambled eggs and sausage. Mom cleaned her plate. I am still in shock. God has his hand in everything that happens in this home and I know that he cleared Mom's head so she could be here fully for Diane's visit.

We spent the morning making plans for Thanksgiving dinner. Mom sat up in bed with pad and pen in hand and made a list of things we will need for Thursday. We even talked about all of us going grocery shopping tomorrow for the extras we will need, to complete the menu. It felt so good to see Mom very much in charge of her home.

She decided to try this new oven potato recipe for her lunch. I was involved in making a chicken salad at the time, but put it on hold when she came in and started stirring her cookpots. When she put her potatoes in the oven, I finished making my chicken salad. I was again amazed to see her eat a portion of her potatoes, some chicken salad and a tomato.

I don't say this lightly, but I feel like I am witnessing a miracle. Mom has required very little extra pain medicine. She is more like her old self. It has been more than a couple of months since I have even had a glimpse of the old Momma. I would guess that I haven't seen Mom like this since the beginning of September. I would have to go back and check my email to be certain. When I altered Mom's pain medicine, I expected her to clear some, but nothing like this. I don't know how long it will last, but Diane and I are enjoying every moment and are giving thanks for each moment that we have with Mom. God was good before Mom cleared, but he really outdid himself with the latest development. Decreasing the medicine helped, but as far as I am concerned, God gets all the credit for what is happening to Mom.

Mom has not answered her phone in a very long time, but she is not only answering her phone, she has made numerous phone calls to friends and family. Janet called to see if she could stop by for a visit with Mom. I had talked to her last week to let her know that Diane would be in town this week and would enjoy a chance to visit with her. She told us she would be stopping by around 4 p.m. I was cooking and the kitchen was not tidy, but she asked that we not worry about trying to straighten it up for her. I was comfortable enough with Janet to relax and not worry. When she arrived, we all gathered in Mom's room. Diane and I were busy telling stories about Mom. Diane shared a photo album that she had put together for Jenny. There was a lot of laughter and warm feelings in that room. Mom told us that she was tired, so we moved to the kitchen to finish our visit.

We got to telling stories about Becky and the strong feeling she has about good customer service. Janet shared the same feelings and very similar tactics in dealing with poor customer service. To me, Becky is kind of like a superhero when it comes to making sure that you get the service that you have paid for. Not to mention, don't anybody consider trying to give any of her family a hard time. Becky may be small, but she is a powerhouse when it involves right and wrong. Consider yourself lucky to have her in your corner.

Janet helped Diane get Mom's Christmas tree out of the box so we could get it set up in Mom's room. We were surprised to see Mom walk into the kitchen. We had been so busy exchanging stories that the time just flew. Janet told us that she probably needed to scoot. What a blessing to have the spiritual support we feel with Janet, not to mention how much fun she is to sit and talk with.

I told Diane later that I wanted us to think about Janet performing Mom's funeral. Mom had expressed interest in Reverend Bennett, but he is retired and I don't know if he would be available to perform the service.

I had prepared a wonderful meal of cranberry chicken, green chili rice and peas. Mom said she was still full from lunch, but she did taste the new recipes I had made. Mom and I watched some of *The Antiques Roadshow*. It was soon time for bed, so Diane and I gathered by her bed to hold hands and say our prayers. Diane and I squeezed each others hands when Mom smiled real big and asked God to bless her "wonderful, funny, bad girls." I would not have traded that moment for anything.

I was ready to hit the sack, but Diane was going to clean up the kitchen and check her email. Diane woke me around 11:30. Mom had not been able to make it to the bathroom in time and Diane did not know how we dealt with times like this. She tells me that I told her how to handle it, but I have very little memory of it. I was so tired from the previous night that I was asleep as soon as my head hit the pillow.

Mom slept until about 6 a.m. I responded to the honk. Mom complained about being cold, so I turned the heat on.

I checked the temperature as I let Grace outside. Folks, it was 35°. Gracie started crooning and bouncing and I broke into a frenzied twist and shout. The cats backed off, but they were talking very loudly to each other. Ringo asked Max what happened if it snowed? Max shook her head and told Ringo that he better brush up on his do-si-do, because it was mandatory participation in square dancing.

Thank you God, for this day so sweet, for Mom's continued alertness and bright spirits, for Mom taking charge of planning for Thanksgiving, for Janet and the comfort and peace she brings into our home, for my Mom's special prayer request concerning her daughters and for a 35° morning. Love, Sue

Green Chili Rice

Great with ham or brisket

1 cup chopped onion

1/4 cup melted butter

4 cups cooked rice

16 oz. small curd cottage cheese

16 oz. sour cream

2 cups grated cheese

2 4 oz. cans chopped green chilies

2/3 tsp salt

1/8 tsp pepper

1/4 cup chopped parsley

    Saute onion in butter

    Combine all ingredients in large casserole

    Mix well

    Bake at 375° for 30 minutes

    Makes 8-12 servings

NOVEMBER 21, 2001

Yesterday was a spectacular day for Mom. She was up early and was ready for her morning toast. Diane started the day as Mom's personal assistant, so to speak. I focused on writing my morning note and later, other assorted tasks that I had wanted to catch up on. Early in the morning, Mom mentioned to Diane that she would give her right arm for a cigarette. When Diane told me this, I responded with, "Why not?" I told Diane that it might mean that Mom might have to use supplemental oxygen at times. The big problem is that I can't be around smoke because it could cause irritation and scarring in my lungs. Diane and I went to talk to Mom about her smoking. She was surprised that we felt she should be able to smoke within certain guidelines. We will move the air purifier to her room. She can only smoke when she is alert and sitting in a chair. I can't be in the room while she smokes. The air purifier should clean out the smoke so that it won't be a problem when I come into her room. Mom got on the phone and called Bryant to ask him to pick up a couple of packs of cigarettes and a lighter. Before I could turn around Bryant was at the door with Mom's smokes. She went to the backdoor and lit her first cigarette. She was surprised that it did not taste as good as she thought, in fact it made her kind of jittery. I was surprised when that turned out to be the only cigarette she smoked Tuesday.

Mom does not have very much time left and if she wishes for something and it is within our power, she will have it. During the day, Diane and I would look at each other and break out into big grins. Mom was back and she came with an attitude. In the future the word "tude" will replace the word attitude. She was on the phone, calling and making all sorts of arrangements. I was so pleased when she told me that she had invited Uncle William and Aunt MM for Thanksgiving lunch. They usually spend Thanksgiving with us, but Mom was doing so poorly that we were trying to keep it very simple. I keep looking at Mom and am overwhelmed with the feeling that we have all been blessed with a miracle from God. I

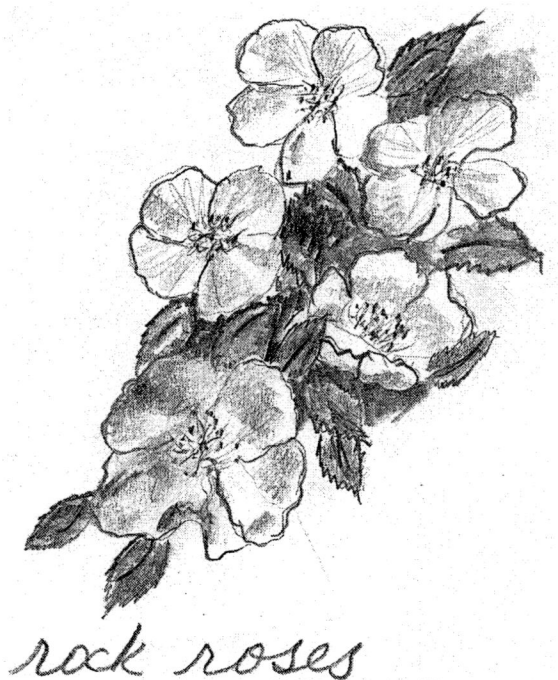

rock roses

143

knew that He had stepped in earlier and gave me the blessing of my health being stable enough that I could take care of all of Mom's needs and wants. Every fiber of my being knows that whenever there is a change and Mom begins to get weaker and closer to death that He will be carrying me through that time. I can't begin to imagine how people go through times like this without complete faith in a loving, generous God.

Uncle William and Aunt MM stopped by and there were animated conversations being exchanged between sister and brother. Sara was in the living room playing Jingle Bells on the piano. Bryant and Jacob had to run an errand and would be back shortly. The whole house felt like it was crackling with the pure energy of love and happiness.

Marianne, the social worker with hospice, came by around 11:30 to visit with all of us. She initially spent time with Diane and me. We talked about how we were enjoying Mom and how bright and alert she is. We also let her know that we know that all of it could change in a heartbeat. I was also relieved to hear Diane tell Marianne how physically challenging she found it was to take care of Mom. She went on to say how it seems like it is something every ten minutes with Mom. I thought I was tired because of my lungs. It felt good to have that kind of feedback. We also talked about how we really need to get together to make Mom's funeral arrangements. It would make it so much easier to do all of that now, rather than waiting till Mom's death. She also spoke to me about having a life outside of caring for Mom. It would be impossible for me to consider doing anything other than running errands, maybe catch a movie or get out for a short while with Lynda. Before Mom got sick, I had decided to volunteer my time as a nurse. If it was only a few hours a week it would be something outside me, this house and Mom. I still plan on doing something like that after Mom is gone.

Kathy arrived soon after Marianne left. Diane had never met Kathy and was impressed. Kathy noticed how Mom's right leg and foot were about two inches larger than her left leg. She called and talked to

Dr. B and got an order for ted hose and Lasix. The ted hose will help reduce the swelling. She was also very impressed with how alert Mom was. She had never seen Mom like she is now.

After Kathy left, I left to go to the grocery store. When I returned, I was met with a frazzled Diane. Mom had her moving plants into the shed and into the house because of the freeze warning. She also had helped Mom whip up a batch of Aunt Lois's roll dough. Mom was just buzzing around the kitchen. A picture had fallen off of Mom's bedroom wall and she wanted some wire to rehang it. She sent Diane into the kitchen to get the needle nose pliers, but Diane was not able to find them fast enough. Diane told me that when she returned to Mom's room, she had the wire cut. Diane told me that she asked Mom how she had managed to cut the wire. I fell out when Diane told me that Mom grinned real big and said, "With my teeth!"

Mom was still glowing bright when we said our prayers and kissed her good night. Diane was in bed by 9 p.m.

It was a 1-honk night. Mom had honked the horn on her walker at 5 a.m., as she was headed for the bathroom. I walked her back to her bed and returned to my bed and dozed lightly. I thought I heard activity in the kitchen. I figured it was Diane up making coffee. WELL- when I walked into the kitchen around 6:30, there was a huge pan with her "fire and ice pickles" in it. Plus, there had been a plate and two cups in the sink that had been washed. I went to check on Mom and she was asleep with the biggest lemon-slice grin on her face. I went and woke Diane so she could share in all of this. Mom had taken 2, 32 ounce jars of dill pickles and cut them in chunks and then made a sweet-hot syrup to cover the pickles. The first thing Becky asked me this morning was if Mom was on prednisone. The answer was no, but she was behaving like she was on a prednisone high.

When I went to let Grace out, I noticed, not only was the temperature 32°, but there was frost on the grass and the bushes. WELL—it was a full-blown foot-tapping, body-twirling and heel-clacking Lord of the Dance routine. Grace was keeping rhythm with her tail. The cats were busy trying to keep their tails out of the clogging. There were joyous hoops from Gracie and me. I was able to tap without the benefit of wearing tap shoes, of course that is something I should talk to my pedicurist about. I am sorry this letter is late, but I had errands. I am just fine. It was a routine visit.

Thank you God, for this day so sweet, for the joy we all feel to experience Mom being Mom, for the surprise of fire and ice pickles, for the comfort of Maryanne's visit, for listening to Sara play Jingle Bells, for the chance to share with Diane this very special and busy time with Mom, for Mom's beautiful smile as she slept and for a glorious frosty morning. Love, Sue

NOVEMBER 22, 2001

Yesterday was another beautiful day for Mom. She was up and stirring cookpots. I was gone most of the day running errands and Diane stayed with Mom. When I returned home, I was pleased to find Marilyn had stopped by for a visit. She was also very impressed with the change in Mom's condition. Diane told me that Mom had her hopping the entire time I was gone. Mom had tried out two new recipes from Irene and Vicky. Mom had finished the stuffing and the candied sweet potatoes for Thanksgiving. She also had prepared a wonderful meatloaf for dinner. She had also prepared this new corn dish with jalapeños and cream cheese. I feel like Mom is possessed with Rambo and Julia Childs at the same time. Mom would take these very short little power naps and would be up into something else. She also has not smoked anymore than that one cigarette. She says that she has no interest. I am sure happy about her decision.

Diane and I said our prayers with Mom and I was asleep by 9:30. Diane says that she was not able to fall asleep till around 1 a.m. Mom honked at about 5 to let me know that she was up and going to the bathroom. She and I both returned to bed. A little later, I heard cabinets opening and closing in the kitchen. Mom had told me that she was going to putter in the kitchen and would honk if she needed me. She was looking forward to alone time in her own kitchen. The feeling of warmth and love swept over me, as I lay curled up in bed. I was savoring every little morsel of the sounds and smells of this Thanksgiving morning. It would not be very long before Becky and Sherri arrived with turkey, dressing, sweet potatoes, cranberry sauce, pumpkin cheesecake and her famous buttermilk fudge. Diane and I scurried around getting the tablecloth on the table and all the other last minute things that have to be done.

It dawned on me that I had not let Grace out. I checked the temperature and it was 35°. It was hokey pokey time. The cats felt like they were too cool to put their little foot in and their little foot out and shake it all about. Grace and I were getting down with the shake it all about part. This home is so rich with blessings. I would have said that before Mom had turned the corner last Sunday.

Becky and Sherri arrived like clockwork around 7:45 carrying all their goodies. Becky had not seen Mom since she has turned this corner. She broke out into a big smile. Sherri gave Mom a big hug. Mom and I had to try the first piece of buttermilk fudge. It will bring a tear to your eye.

Thank you God, for this day so sweet, for Mom's continued gift of vigor and enthusiasm, for Diane's humor and how she has stepped right up and been there 100 percent for Mom, for Becky and Diane who have pulled together to give me the free time that I so desperately needed and for this day that we can all come together to give thanks for our many blessings. Love, Sue

Fire and Ice Pickles

1 gallon sliced dill pickles

3 Tbs hot sauce

6 cups sugar

1 tsp dry red pepper

6 cloves garlic

> Drain brine off pickles and discard
>
> Mix ingredients well and stir into drained pickles
>
> Mix well
>
> Pack into a one gallon jar (the one the pickles came out of)
>
> Refrigerate
>
> Shake once or twice for two days

NOVEMBER 23, 2001

Yesterday was a wondrous day for all. Mom was up early preparing the last minute dishes that go with the turkey. We were all surprised that this red cabbage dish turned out to have a great taste. Diane and I were worried, since Mom had run out of cider vinegar and we had completely run out of sugar. Mom called Bryant and he will stop by the store before he comes for Thanksgiving dinner.

Becky and Sherri arrived early in the morning carrying the turkey, sweet potatoes, cranberries, gravy, pumpkin cheesecake and butter milk fudge. I think I wrote something very similar to this list of dishes, but it bears repeating. Becky ran the vacuum quickly and then washed and styled Mom's hair. It felt good to have all the sisters together. Becky and Sherri could not stay long because Sherri was having to work at Garden Ridge Pottery and Becky needed to finish up her Thanksgiving meal for her home.

Uncle William, Aunt MM and Lee arrived early. Aunt MM, Diane and I worked as a team getting the roll dough rolled out and cut. The relish tray needed to be arranged, along with seasoning the green beans. Mom and Uncle William were both sound asleep in Mom's bedroom. Mom was taking a well-earned nap. She had not only finished up several side dishes, but had gotten cleaned up and put on some snazzy pajamas. Bryant, Jacob and Sara soon arrived with the much needed sugar and vinegar.

We all gathered together and gave thanks for the love of family and the love that went into preparing all the wonderful food. We also said an extra prayer of thanksgiving for Mom being able to participate and enjoy all that Thanksgiving is.

After everybody left, Aunt MM and I cleaned up the kitchen. Mom, Diane and Lee were all asleep. Uncle William wasn't far from joining them in a nap. Bryant was helping with collecting all the garbage and the kids were watching TV. It wasn't too very long before everybody left to go home and continue their naps. Diane woke up and we watched a movie together. Mom was awake soon with some breakthrough pain. It was not too long before we got it under control. Mom only wanted a couple of rolls toasted for dinner. I don't know how long Diane stayed awake, because I poured myself in bed at 9 p.m. and fell fast asleep.

It was a 1-honk night, with some 5 a.m. hammering thrown in. When I heard the hammering I was petrified that Mom had fallen and was banging on the cabinet to get some help. I found her hammering on some ice that fits into her ice crusher. I had never shown her how she could release the circle of ice, without having to take a hammer and an ice pick to it. I got her ice shaved and walked her back to her bed. She told me I was excused because she could tuck herself in just fine. I returned to bed and watched an old movie.

I was disappointed to find it 63° this morning. It felt cooler than that when I opened the door. It had evidently rained during the night. I did give the cats a hard look to see if I could detect anything that might indicate tampering with the thermometer. I told them that they were off of the hook now, but I would be keeping a close eye on them.

Thank you God, for this day so sweet, for the early morning sounds and smells that told me Mom was doing what she loved doing the most, for Becky's buttermilk fudge, for Sherri making time in her busy schedule to come and see her Granny, for Bryant saving us from a sugar shortage, for all of us being able to come together to give thanks to you for all of our many blessings and for Jenny, who remained at home to care for her dad and all the critters so her mom could be here to share this last Thanksgiving with her Mother, and I am also thankful that Jenny took a step of faith and prepared her first Thanksgiving meal, all on her own. As far as I am concerned every day is going to be a day of thanksgiving. Love, Sue

Buttermilk Fudge

2 cups sugar

1 tsp soda

1 cup pecans

1 cup buttermilk

3 Tbs butter

    Combine sugar and buttermilk in a saucepan

    Bring to a rolling boil

    Add soda and butter

    Cook to medium ball stage (245°)

    Remove from heat

    Add nuts

    Beat until slightly cool

    Do not over beat

    Will harden fast

    Drop by spoon onto waxed paper

NOVEMBER 24, 2001

Mom had another wonderful day yesterday. She was awake early in anticipation of a visit from her Sister FiFi, Uncle Dade and Stephen. They arrived around 10:15. I was so glad that Aunt FiFi and Stephen would have a chance to enjoy Mom's energy. None of us know how long it will last. Soon after they arrived, Vicky arrived to make Mom's bed. Babe and Francis arrived right after Vicky got here. The house was filling up. Mom started talking about getting barbecue and making this new recipe with corn and cream cheese. Diane would come and ask me about the barbecue and I told her to try and persuade Mom to wait till later, because nobody wanted lunch. Well, Bryant, Jacob and Sara arrived and before I knew it he turned around and left to get barbecue. Uncle William, Aunt MM and Lee arrived. By the time Bryant got back with the barbecue, Babe and Francis had left. I peeked in Mom's room and Mom was sitting up in bed eating a big plate of barbecue, potato salad and corn. As it turns out, she was the one really craving the barbecue meal and if others wanted to eat, that was ok.

Stephen showed us some professional photographs he had made with Sammy (hope that is the right spelling), his beautiful black cat. Sammy became ill with some type of kidney disease and did not survive. The pictures are a comfort to Stephen. I really need to look into getting some professional pictures done with Grace. Stephen also helped with getting my new computer set up on my desk. There was a major tangle of cords and wires. He very calmly sorted it all out and I had a beautiful setup with monitor, keyboard and my "Burbie."

Kathy arrived to do her assessment on Mom. I took her around and she met all of the family. She was so good natured about all of the family and the introductions. It was important to me that she meet the people that love Mom. Mom's swelling in her legs was still pretty significant. Kathy also heard some crackles in the bases of Mom's lungs. She felt like the lasix would clear the crackles up. Bryant and the kids left to go ice skating. Stephen was taking pictures of Mom, Diane and me. I had tried my hand earlier with the video camera and had little success. Our home was so full of laughter, old stories being remembered and love and the spirit of gratitude for our many blessings. It was soon time for the Denton-type relatives to leave. Stephen will have to fly out of Dallas Saturday, so he can meet with some coworkers to continue on with a business trip. Diane walked Uncle William to his car. They were talking about a problem that has come up with where Mom will be buried. I will go into that issue at a later time.

We all took a short nap after all of our family had left for home. I got up and decided to do a little Christmas shopping while Diane was here. It was so nice to get out and listen to Christmas music on the radio and buy the first gifts of the season. It was dark when I returned home and Mom was taking a nap. It was not very long before she was awake and wanted to play a game of Skip-Bo. Before we played the cards, there was this unnecessary control struggle with Mom's scheduled pain medicine. She is so quick to jump on me flat-footed, when it comes to anything surrounding her medicine. In fact, when I left the room, she turned to Diane for support. Diane told her that she would have done the same thing. Mom told her that, "Well, you can too."

I know Mom is frightened about how strong her medicine is, but she can't just stop it completely. She went into the kitchen and cooked herself some oatmeal. I whispered to Diane that she needed a lactaid to keep her from getting a belly ache. Mom quietly took her lactaid. After she calmed down and I took a deep breath, we played a game of Skip-Bo. I beat Mom by one card. She was ready to turn in for the night. We all said our prayers and kissed her goodnight. I was ready for bed, but felt very sad when I thought about how little time there is left of Diane's visit. I jokingly told her that I was happy that Mom was back with her spurs on, but it could be painful at times. Diane told me that it was ok to say "ouch" when someone had spurred you. She told Mom about the spurs story and Mom just laughed.

It was a 2-honk night, with a third honk being imagined by myself.

Thank you God, for this day so sweet, for joyous family gatherings, for good barbecue, for Christmas music, for the game of Skip-Bo with Mom and for the gift of Diane as my sister who brings me such comfort in these sad and confusing times. Love, Sue

NOVEMBER 25, 2001

Mom had a very nice day yesterday. We started the morning slow. Before we knew it Uncle William and Aunt MM were here to say good bye to Diane. They were still talking about how much they enjoyed Thanksgiving. As they were leaving Becky and Tom arrived. They were coming to visit and not to clean or repair anything. Becky brought some more of her buttermilk fudge. Tom had his new digital camera that he had gotten for his birthday on the twenty-third. Becky did give me a wonderful haircut while she was here. Mostly there was a lot of animated conversations going on. Towards the end of their visit, Tom took pictures of Mom and her three daughters. Diane and Becky were all trying to stand behind me, so parts of them would be hidden from the camera. Mom just shook her head. Before we knew it, Becky and Tom had to leave. They were going to look at carpet. Sherri had to work and that is why she had not been able to come along.

Diane worked on packing and decided to take a quick nap before loading the car for the trip home. I kept telling myself that she would be back in a couple of weeks. I was also concerned about her upcoming surgery to put stents in the arteries going to her legs. She has peripheral vascular disease and her legs get really tired from having a reduced blood flow. It is a pretty standard surgery, but it is still surgery.

After Diane's nap, she got up and hooked up Mom's VCR to her TV. She also spent some quiet time with her Mother. I put on my portable tank and helped Diane load her car. It was time for Diane to leave. Diane told Mom to be easy with me. Mom said she would try. Diane kissed her good bye and I walked her to the front porch. We hugged each other and held on tight a little longer than usual. I did not start to cry until she turned to wave good bye to me. For a few moments I felt so young and overwhelmed with what lay before me. It was such a gift to have Diane here 24/7. I could have done it by myself, but I had the chance to share the care with Diane. She did such an outstanding job. I wiped my tears and went in to check on Mom. We comforted each other. Mom wanted to take a nap and I went in to do some catalog shopping. Mom and I would not be able to relax until we got a phone call from Diane telling us that she was home and safe. We got that call at 9:15.

Mom and I said our prayers and turned in for the night. It was a 2-honk night. At 5 a.m. I thought I heard Ringo in the kitchen and went to check on things. I found Mom with her head in the refrigerator. She told me that she was hungry. She thought a fried egg sandwich with a slice of tomato would taste good. She went back to bed and I made her sandwich and a cup of hot chocolate.

I went to let Grace out and the thermometer was broken, so I used my internal thermometer to guide my way. Well, I could see my breath and Grace's breath. I performed an inspired hula. The cats questioned my choice of dance, but then they question everything.

Thank you God, for this day so sweet, for the gift of Tom's picture-taking, for a Becky haircut, for that extra-long hug and for delivering Diane safely home. Love, Sue

NOVEMBER 26, 2001
The Baxters are Diane's in-laws

What a wonderful day Sunday was for Mom. She woke up bright-eyed and bushy tailed. She sat in her recliner and watched a church service on TV and then read the Sunday paper. She did not just glance at it like she has in the past, but she really read it from front to back. She talked to me about how she wanted to help me bake a gingerbread house for Christmas. It has been a while since I have made one. Needless to say, I was thrilled at the thought of us creating a masterpiece. We continued talking about what we could cook and freeze, in planning ahead for the Christmas visit with the Baxter's. Mom and I are pleased to find out that Jenny's boyfriend Billy is going to be able to be here for Christmas. I was so pleased to see Mom have an appetite. She snacked every couple of hours through the day.

Uncle William and Aunt MM stopped by for their Sunday afternoon visit. They are basking in the glow that emanates from Mom. After their visit, Mom spent some time organizing her address book. She has not looked at it since August. She had a pleasant interruption when Barbara, a childhood friend, called to visit with her. It is wonderful that Mom has remained in contact with some of her childhood friends. Diane and Jenny also called to check in on Mom.

Mom and I got ourselves all excited and wound up when we talked about their upcoming visit. Late in the afternoon, our good friend and neighbor, Pat, stopped by for a visit. Before Pat had left, we were surprised when Lynda and Kelly stopped by for a visit. We had not seen them since before Thanksgiving because they had been helping Kelly's daughter, Melissa, move into her new home. They had wonderful new stories about Andrew and all the new things he has learned to do. Before they left, Lisa and Dria, our next door neighbors came for a visit. Dria is about two and a half years old and Lisa is expecting another baby in the spring. Dria entertained us with her piano playing. We were surprised to look up and realize that it was 8 p.m. It was Dria's bedtime.

Mom and I talked about what a wonderfully full day it had been. We said our prayers and exchanged goodnight kisses.

It was a 4-honk night. Mom really did not need me to help her, but she had promised that she would honk if she needed to go to the bathroom.

At 5 a.m. Mom honked for me. I laughed out loud when I discovered that Mom had been up and fixed herself a tossed salad. She said that she did not need my help to go to the bathroom, but she was keeping her promise regarding the honking. I gave her a hug and a kiss and returned to bed to catch an extra forty winks.

Thank you God, for this day so sweet, for a Sunday full of friends and family, for Church services on TV, for the warm feelings associated with menu planning with Mom and for the laughter that came with that 5 a.m. honk. Love, Sue

NOVEMBER 27, 2001

The days keep getting better and better. Mom was up early, which had been her habit before she had gotten so sick. When I say up, I mean up doing things not just laying in bed. Vicky arrived early to help Mom with her bath and bed. Vicky just looked on in amazement at the varied collection of wild Christmas socks that Becky had bought Mom. I had gotten her a pair that had a crown on the ankle and the word Princess above it. Mom told Vicky that she did not know why her children were standing in line to do such nice things for her. Vicky responded, "That is easy, they love you and want to spoil you and I don't mean spoil in a bad way!" Before Vicky left, Margaret came by for a visit. She brought the most beautiful greenery with bright red berries. I put the branches in a white milk glass pitcher. The arrangement filled Mom's room up with Christmas beauty from the garden. They had an animated visit and are making plans to get together soon.

I had fixed egg salad for lunch and Mom cleaned her plate. She was busy making her lists and she was checking them twice, I assure you. The lists are about groceries for this week, groceries for Christmas baking, groceries for when the Baxters come for Christmas, lists of gifts that she is planning on giving at Christmas and "things to do" lists for me. I find myself wearing the biggest grin as I write about all of this. There is certainly a vibrant kind of energy to be found in this home.

Mom spent the afternoon reading through cooking magazines, Christmas catalogs and Guideposts. She would hop up every now and then and rummage through her pantry or the freezer. I listen for a problem, but I don't run in each time that I hear Mom up. In the first place, it irritates her, and I most definitely don't want to irritate her. Secondly, she is really very stable with her walker. She needs some space where I am not hovering over her. I welcome the chance to step back and enjoy watching her reclaim her home.

Lynda came over for a moment to leave some turkey hash for dinner and to borrow our leaf blower. She and Mom took some time to catch up on what was happening in her home. I spent most of the day doing odd chores and keeping a steady flow of shaved ice going in Mom's direction. Shaved ice is her favorite thing to munch on, not to mention its calming influence on dry heaves.

After dinner we watched *The Antique Roadshow*. After the show, I decided to talk to Mom about honking for me during the night. I told her that I wanted her to honk for me if she felt unsteady or needed any kind of help. If she felt safe enough, then I was ok with her going to the bathroom by herself. She was very pleased with that kind of arrangement. It was soon time for our prayers and goodnight kiss. Mom did have a restless night. She did not honk for me, but Grace had awakened me a couple of times so she could go outside. Each time, I found Mom doing something. She told me that she had slept, but woke up and did not want to stay in bed. She had been down to the den, looking through scraps of material. When I got up at 5, she had pulled together all the ingredients for chili and for okra, peas and tomatoes. She had also fixed herself a cup of hot chocolate.

When I got up to let Grace out at 5, I knew that the temperature was 42° with the wind-chill in the low thirties. It was "Cotton Eyed Joe" time. Ringo was puzzled because I was wanting him to join in, but it wasn't snowing. Max had told him to be ready to swing his partner when it snowed, but it wasn't mandatory participation today. I thought that the volume of their collective sigh of relief was a little excessive. Grace and I did well on our own.

Thank you God, for this day so sweet, for having a mother that enjoys how different each of her children are, for shaved ice and for shared hot chocolate with my mom on a cold November morning. Love, Sue

NOVEMBER 28, 2001

Mom spent yesterday reclaiming her kitchen. She emptied the dishwasher and moved some bowls and pans back to where they were before she got sick. I had moved some things around in the cabinets when I was cooking and cleaning. I was so mesmerized by watching her move around the kitchen that she would look at me and say, "Why are you staring at me! Stop it!" I would apologize and try to explain that it was like being able to take a breath, watching sunrise after I had been told that I would never see another. The only way I could stop staring was to leave the room. I would return for a few minutes at a time. She was whipping up a wonderful chili in honor of the cold weather. Mom also decided that she was hungry for okra, tomatoes and peas, so she pulled out her cooking pots. She reacquainted herself with her pantry. She spent some time putting cans of soup, bags of dried beans and boxes of rice back where she felt they belonged. I could almost swear that I saw her caress a bag of stuffing mix. She was truly home as she was surrounded by her kitchen.

Lynda was coming over to stay with Mom so I could run to the store. Marilyn surprised me with a call, asking if she could come over and visit. Mom was excited about Lynda and Marilyn coming over. She said that they were two of her most favorite friends and were always welcome. Lynda had also come to help me cover the outdoor faucets. We looked for buckets to put over the faucets. Lynda went out to cover the faucets and discovered that they were already wrapped with insulation foam. That was a big "oops" on my part. Lynda demonstrated her feelings about all of this by putting my head in a headlock. One never gets too old for classic wrestling holds.

Marilyn soon arrived and Lynda was going to go home and Marilyn was going to stay with Mom. Marilyn brought wonderful homemade cheese soup for Mom. Before I could leave, Mom started having dry heaves. Marilyn got Mom's bucket for her to hold and Lynda got her shaved ice. I saw things were under control, so I left to go shopping.

I really enjoyed the combination of the icy cold temperature and listening to Christmas music on the car radio. I was surprised at how many people were at the grocery store. I guess they were putting in supplies for the cold weather. When I got home, Marilyn told me that Kathy had been by to check on Mom. I also found this beautiful Christmas cactus that I thought had died, on the table. Diane had put it in the shed when she was here and when Lynda and I were looking for buckets we found this cactus in full bloom. While I was gone, Lynda brought it in and Marilyn cleaned it up. How rich Mom and I are to have friends that will weather the cold to bring soup, protect our pipes and clean up a cactus.

Marilyn needed to scoot home before the weather got any worse. Mom was excited when I told her that I had picked up several "Taste of Home" cooking magazines. She did not waste any time in devouring them. I started to put up the groceries and before very long Mom joined me in the kitchen. She wanted to clean out the refrigerator. Mom pulled up a chair in front of the refrigerator and started to rearrange, throw away and combine like items. She was in heaven and I was too. It was truly a "one small step" moment. All she had to do now was just give me a look to interrupt my stare. She had cheese soup for dinner and I enjoyed her chili. We watched a little TV and turned in for the night.

Mom didn't honk for me during the night.

When I went to let Grace out at 5 a.m., I noticed that it was raining and it was 33°. The news had said the wind-chill was in the teens. I broke into an inspired Indian Dance for snow. I heard Ringo ask Max if this was a good time for prayer. Max suggested that they also say the rosary and fast, in addition to the prayers. I don't think they are praying for snow. Love, Sue

NOVEMBER 29, 2001

Mom had a full day yesterday. Vicky came early to assist Mom with her bath. Mom is so comfortable with Vicky. They spent most of their time talking about favorite recipes. After Vicky left, Mom took a large dose of lasix. Her legs are so swollen. As the morning progressed, the Lasix was working overtime, leaving Mom feeling washed out. It only slowed her down a little bit. She decided to make a spicy zucchini soup. Lynda was going to bring the Italian sausage and beef broth that we needed for the soup. Linda came by and offered to go get chili dogs for lunch. Mom was content with her mug of navy bean soup. After Lynda returned and we ate our hot dogs, I felt like wrapping myself up in a quilt and taking a nap. Lynda told me that Mom was asleep and she was going to go home and let me curl up and take a nap. I surprised myself by dozing off for about thirty minutes.

Mom was awake and we decided to make this big pot of soup. Working side by side with Mom, in her warm cozy kitchen, surrounded with wonderful aromas, was a piece of heaven on earth. I imagined it was like how a cat feels when he is surrounded with some good catnip. I had to fight the impulse to get frisky and roll around on the floor. I was most definitely purring.

Mom went to lay down, while the soup simmered for two hours and I kept track of the weather. I do love the cold and the idea of snow is great, but cold and wet means that I don't breathe as well. The dry cold feels good to me.

Mom was up and down in the late afternoon. The lasix was beginning to wear off. I was able to finish up some Christmas shopping, using catalogs. It does require a step of faith to trust that your orders will arrive in time for Christmas. I am just about to wind up my shopping, which feels wonderful. I will have a few things that I will have to pick up, but not many.

Mom ate a pretty good dinner and was ready to turn in early for the night. When we said our prayers, we said an extra prayer for Diane. She is having stents placed in the arteries in her legs to help improve the blood flow on Thursday afternoon.

It was a 1-honk night. Grace did wake me at 5 a.m. and led me to the kitchen where Mom was making another pot of chili. I started chuckling at the whole picture. Grace evidently thought that something was amiss to wake me up and point out Mom to me. She was not asking to go out, but she wanted me to know that she was on top of things. This is why we call her "the night nurse." I did insist that Grace go on out and do her morning thing.

I was pleased to find the temperature at 30° and the wind chill at 17°. The cats went into hiding under the table, as Grace began to howl as I began my interpretation of a Highland Fling. I have never danced a Highland Fling, but that did not stop me this morning. Ringo asked Max if there were any saints that protected cats in these circumstances. Max told Ringo that it would be worth researching.

Thank you God, for this day so sweet, for sharing a foot long chili dog with my best friend on a cold winter day, for the whole zucchini soup experience with Mom, for the chance to be able to do my Christmas shopping in the comfort of my room, for the watchful eye of the night nurse and for the peace and comfort that comes with prayer. Love, Sue

NOVEMBER 30, 2001

Mom had a nice day yesterday. She started it early, by making a big pot of chili. A little later I went to put a pie in the oven and found a pork chop casserole in there. Initially, Mom denied any knowledge of this and I denied having anything to do with it. A few moments later she called me back to her room and told me that she had a vague recollection of preparing the pork chops earlier. She smiled and asked me what she was going to do about this "sleepcooking" that she is doing now. My response was that we will be busy eating.

We talked to Diane on the phone several times before she left to go to the hospital. Jenny will be with her. We spent the day puttering around the house. We had Diane's surgery on our mind and tried to keep occupied to make the time pass. Mom did some reading, visited with friends on the phone and made lists of grocery items that she would need to do her Christmas baking.

After lunch, she asked me to help her sit on the floor in front of the pots and pans cabinet. She was going to arrange the pots to suit her. I spent some time playing with these special glasses that Kelley gave me. They are similar to the type of glasses you wear when watching a 3-D movie. With my Christmas glasses, it somehow makes lights take on a snowflake kind of shape, with a beautiful soft glow. Mom and I both played with them. Kelly knows the kinds of things one needs to intensify the Christmas experience. She is my kind of friend. During the day Mom kept me busy making shaved ice for her. I bought a Hawaii shaved ice machine in July before her throat surgery. I thought that it would feel soothing to her throat. She really did not ask for any shaved ice, until the last couple of months. She now consumes large quantities of shaved ice daily. Mom says that it is one of the most satisfying experiences she has discovered. It is a wonderful way for her to keep hydrated.

I did a little more catalog Christmas shopping. I think Mom and I will work on Christmas cards Friday. Both of us enjoy doing the Christmas cards each year. Jenny called before dinner to let us know that Diane was out of surgery and was doing well. She will be out of the hospital today. Bryant also called and talked to Mom for a while. Jacob and Sara are doing great in school.

Mom and I turned in early for the night. At 9:30 I found Mom in the kitchen making herself a bacon sandwich. It feels so good watching Mother begin to eat again. The snacks are small portions, but they are frequent.

It was a 1-honk night. We were all up around 5:30.

The temperature was 32°. It was Salsa dancing time. The cats asked Grace again how long winter lasted. Grace was very matter of fact when she told them that winter was not the problem, it was the combination of winter and Christmas that posed the greater risk of mandatory participation in song and dance. Grace asked Ringo and Max if they had tried on their different Christmas getups. They asked for Grace to clarify what she meant by "getups." Grace explained that she had a Santa hat and Santa beard, antlers, sweaters and a jinglebell collar. I did hear Ringo ask Grace if I accepted a doctor's note excusing him from participation. Grace just smiled and shook her head no.

Thank you God, for this day so sweet, for Mom's inspired cooking adventures, for the comfort that prayer offered us as we waited on news concerning Diane's surgery, for shaved ice, for friends that knew you were in need of magic Christmas glasses and for Christmas cards that announce the miracle of your birth. Love, Sue

DECEMBER 2, 2001

Mom had a full day yesterday. She started early, as this has become her routine. She had started to make her toast and I offered to finish it and bring it to her bed.

Becky and Sherri arrived early carrying bags of groceries and secret Christmas presents. The Christmas that Mom ordered is coming to Becky's address, so it can be kept secret. Sherri started right away with putting up the groceries and taking out the trash. She was a big help to me and I had lots of hugs for her. Carol arrived right after Becky and Sherri arrival. Carol had brought Mom the most wonderful wooden Santa and teddy bear. The bear is in honor of Mom's nickname at school, which was "Momma Bear." Carol had interesting stories to tell about her recent jury duty experience. Mom really enjoyed her visit with Carol.

After Carol left, I started getting ready to go and run a few errands while Becky and Sherri were at home with Mom. I had to exchange a three-foot pre-lit tree because half the lights weren't working. When I returned home Becky had the house spit spot, Mom's hair washed and styled and all the Christmas decorations down from the attic. She is an amazing woman. Becky was eager to go home and see her new carpet. She and Tom had their whole house recarpeted.

Mom took a short nap after they left and I sat in front of my air conditioner with my oxygen on high. There was something in the air that was making it difficult for anyone with lung problems to breathe. Mom even asked to have her oxygen put on.

Mom and I turned in early. She honked for me later, so she could tell me that Uncle Dade had been taken to the hospital with shortness of breath. We said an extra prayer for the Spark's family. Mom honked for me twice during the night.

Thank you God, for this day so sweet, for all of the hard work Becky and Sherri did on Saturday, for the surprise visit from Carol and for the excitement that comes with Christmas secrets. Love, Sue

DECEMBER 3, 2001

Well, this is my second try. I had gotten down to the last few words and there was a power outage and I lost it all. So, if this is a little shorter than usual, I hope you understand. Mom had a wonderfully full day yesterday. Mom started very early. Grace, the night nurse, woke me to let me know that Mom was in the kitchen making toast, oatmeal and hot chocolate. Grace cracks me up with her tattling. She is such a wonderful old mother hen.

Aunt FiFi called to let us know about Uncle Dade. He is intensive care and has been diagnosed with pneumonia. The doctor doesn't think it necessary to have Stephen and Susanne come home. That statement is certainly hopeful, but I am sure that times like these make it so difficult to live so far away from home. We will be holding the Spark's family close in prayer.

Mom and I talked about what we would like to accomplish. I needed to work on installing my printer. Diane offered the technical phone support. Mom wanted to work on hemming some dresses. I also had begun to pull out the Christmas ornaments for the tree. First, there was church on TV that was watched and then Mom had the Sunday newspaper to slowly read. Mom's old friend, Mildred, called to catch up on the activities here in Dallas. Mom looks forward to her Sunday calls from Mildred. I put some pork chops in the crockpot and made my favorite green chili rice dish for our dinner later in the afternoon. Bryant, Jacob and Sara stopped by for a visit. Bryant had some clothes getting washed at the local Laundromat. Sara helped put some ornaments on the tree. They were not able to stay long because they had plans to attend a Christmas concert later in the evening. Before Mom and I had dinner our neighbor, Mrs. Ramsey, came by with baked custard, vegetable soup and chili mac casserole. We are certainly blessed with generous and caring neighbors.

It was not very long before it was time to turn in for the night. Mom was restless last night, so it was a 3-honk night. The temperature left me uninspired this morning.

Thank you God, for this day so sweet, for the news that Uncle Dade was stable, for Bryant, Jacob and Sara's visit, and for neighbors like Mrs. Ramsey. Love, Sue

DECEMBER 4, 2001

Mom was not feeling very well yesterday, but it did not stop her from accomplishing the goals that she had set for herself. Mom's mind set is that if she keeps pushing forward with different tasks she might get to feeling better. When I am feeling under the weather, I don't automatically jump into projects with the thought that it will cure my ills. Mom has always responded with work in an attempt to cure what ails her. Mom reminded me of a small toddler that would play real hard then suddenly fall fast asleep, sleep for a short period of time and then wake and pick up where she had left off.

I spoke with Diane, about having trouble keeping up with Mom. Here she is in hospice, on heavy narcotics and now relies on a walker to get around, and I am barely keeping up with her. Yesterday was difficult for me with all the moisture in the air. I was able to just barely keep up with her. The first thing I accomplished in the morning was decorating the Christmas tree in Mom's room. Mom spent a lot of time in the morning, working on her sewing machine. She finally called Lisa, from next door, to see if she could identify what the problem was with the needle. Before it was all over with, Lisa's husband, Joe, was here along with Dria and Grace, the little girl that Lisa takes care of during the day. Dria, Grace and I played the piano and named the different things that we saw on the tree. Joe did his part with the sewing machine and Lisa tried to help Mom with putting a machine hem in a dress. Lisa wasn't happy with the stitch, so she took the dress home to work on it. Mom didn't see anything wrong with the stitch, so she put a hem in another dress she had basted.

After Mom finished her lunch, she decided it was time to make a chocolate coke cake. We could not find the cocoa. I thought that might put a halt to that project and she could rest a little. I realized that I had a momentary lapse in thinking, because Mom got on the phone and talked with our neighbor, Pat, and arranged for her to drop off some cocoa. Pat soon arrived with the cocoa and had Grace's Christmas present. She had a Santa hat and a furry candy cane for her to play with. Grace is so patient with me when I try on different costumes on her. She did strike a few poses for the cats. I thought Ringo was going to faint when he saw Grace wearing her Santa hat. I heard him mumble to himself, "It is true about Christmas outfits! What has happened to her rule book about what cats do and don't do!" Max reminded him that I was one of those people that don't believe in coloring inside the lines.

After Pat left, Mom began cooking and mixing up the ingredients for her cake. I started fixing our dinner. Mom wanted a bacon, fried egg and tomato sandwich. I put the cake in the oven and felt overwhelmed when I looked at the kitchen. I initially told myself that I could clean it up tomorrow. I started puttering around and put on some Christmas music and before I knew it the kitchen was clean and I had put quite a few more ornaments on the tree.

At bedtime Mom and I talked about the day's activities. She told me that she felt like the day was a success, because she did not let not feeling well keep her from accomplishing the goals that she had set for her day. I felt comforted by her comments. Mom has always been a wonderful example of how hard work pays off. She is most certainly not looking for an excuse to stay in bed and be waited on hand and foot. She has always welcomed a challenge.

As we said our prayers, I included an extra prayer of thanks for being able to witness how Mom embraced the challenges that she was faced with during the day.

Mom honked for me twice during the night and Grace woke me to let me know that it was 4 a.m. and Mom was in the kitchen baking sweet potatoes. I asked her if she needed any help and she told me to go back to bed. I got up at 5 to check on Mom and found that she had a roast in the slow cooker, a ham and rice casserole and a beef and beans casserole ready for the freezer. She also was in the process of candying the sweet potatoes. Oh, she had also made the frosting for the coke cake. I asked her if she was feeling any better this morning. She told me that she was not sure, but it felt good to get some of the cooking out of the way.

Thank you God, for this day so sweet, for the gift of watching Mom accomplish her goals for the day, for good neighbors, for the comfort from favorite family recipes, for the inspiration that comes when listening to your Christmas music and for Grace, the night nurse, and her continued vigilance in caring for Mom. Love, Sue

Coke Cake

2 cups all purpose flour

2 cups sugar

1 tsp soda

1 cup coca cola

1 cup butter

2 Tbs cocoa

½ cup buttermilk

2 eggs beaten

1 tsp vanilla

1 ½ cups miniature marshmallows

1 cup finely chopped pecans

Combine flour and soda, set aside
Combine coke, butter and cocoa in heavy saucepan
Bring to a boil, stirring constantly
Gradually stir into flour mixture
Stir in buttermilk, eggs, vanilla, and marshmallows
Pour in a greased and floured 13 x 9 pan
Bake at 350° for 30 minutes

Coke frosting

½ cup butter
6 Tbs coca cola
3 Tbs cocoa
1 16 ounce package powdered sugar
1 tsp vanilla
Bring butter, coke and cocoa to a boil over medium heat, stirring until butter melts
Remove from heat
Stir in powdered sugar, vanilla extract
Add pecans
Spread over warm cake

DECEMBER 5, 2001

Yesterday was a very restless day for Mom. She felt like she was sleep-walking. That is what it looked liked. Mom had a glazed look in her eyes that reminded me of what it looked like when she was over medicated. Mom would lay down for a few minutes and then hop up and go address Christmas cards or cook something. Yesterday she had cooked all those casseroles early in the morning. As a psychiatric nurse, I would have described her as agitated. I spent most of the day following Mom around. I was able to finish decorating Mom's tree and our Christmas tree. They really are magical. I have to get my Santa collection out, along with my North Pole Village.

Kathy came by to do Mom's assessment. She is going to have a podiatrist to come out and check out a painful ingrown toenail that Mom has. While she was here, she suggested that I give Mom an Ativan. I reluctantly did so. Mom has been known to behave in an odd manner after she takes an Ativan. She proceeded to fulfill my prediction regarding her behavior. I did collect all the pain medicine. I told Mom that I think she has inadvertently taken extra medicine. From now on, I will dispense all pain medicine.

When we said our prayers I said an extra prayer that she would begin to clear up mentally.

It was a 3-honk night. I was relieved when I looked in her eyes early this morning and they no longer looked like they were glazed. I think that she is on her way to being her old self.

Thank you God, for this day so sweet, for the memories associated with all of the Christmas ornaments and for Mom's clear eyes this morning. Love, Sue

DECEMBER 6, 2001

Mom's head began to clear yesterday from what I think was her being over medicated. I was so very relieved to see her brighten up and she was not so restless. Unfortunately, Mom woke up with a very painful left heel. She was not able to tolerate any weight on it, so getting around was slow going for her. I put my nursing cap on and thought about what would be some of the most obvious problems with her left heel. The most obvious would be a flare up of arthritis or an inflamed Achilles' tendon. A non-steroidal, anti-inflammatory medicine is what would probably help to relieve the inflammatory process. The only glitch is that Mom can't take aspirin since she had her whipple surgical procedure. I put in a call to Kathy so I could get some feedback from her or Dr. B. Kathy agreed with my assessment and will let me know if Dr. B. recommends anything different.

Mom spent most of the morning working on our Christmas cards. She also had her head in her cookbooks. Lynda came by to give me a hand with putting up empty ornament boxes, helping me find my Santa collection and also carried bags of trash to the alley. Catalog shopping is sure handy, but you are left with the boxes and packing papers to dispose of. We did take some time and shared lunch and girl talk, which we both really enjoyed. It is hard to believe that Andrew is already one year old. Time does pick up speed as you get older. When I am feeling really alone and am surrounded by rampaging Indians, I know that when Lynda comes over, I am able to get in touch with my problem solving abilities and I find the strength to fight off hoards of wild Indians.

Uncle William called to give us an update on Uncle Dade's condition. He is still in ICU and does not seem to be responding to the antibiotics as well as they had hoped. Stephen and Susanne are both flying in Wednesday so they can see their Dad and give their Mom a chance to catch up on some much needed rest. Uncle William was tearful as he talked about his concern for his sister and Dade. He was comforted when I told him that Mom seemed to be having a better day.

Mom was able to take a nap after lunch. I spent some time sorting through Christmas decorations. I have not located the wreaths for the doors. I am left weak in the knees with the thought that they could be in the den closet. You need to have your affairs in order, along with your next of kin notification, to go into that closet.

When Mom woke, I told her about Uncle Dade and we bowed our heads in prayer. Mom was wanting to do some Christmas baking, but we did not have the ingredients and she could not improvise this time. I suggested that she focus on keeping her foot up and let it calm down, before she decides to cook. She quickly dismissed that idea. In my bones, I know that she will conjure up something in the kitchen before the day is over.

The mail brought lots of Christmas packages. One of the packages held an early Christmas present for me. I decided that I could not live without this computer accessory, so I gave myself a present. You will never guess, so I will tell you. I am the proud owner of a set of plastic, hot pink Cadillac fins, with adhesive, to attach them to the sides of my computer. If anyone else is interested in making a statement, I can connect you with my source. After Mom and I had dinner, Janet called to set a time to come by for a visit on Thursday. Mom and I are looking forward to her visit.

Mom and I said our prayers and we turned in early for the night. She honked for me around 11:30 and told me that she wanted me to walk her to the bathroom. Around 2:45 I heard a loud thump and came tearing out of my bed. Gracie had the lead as we checked the bathroom and Mom's room. Mom was awake and she did not know what had caused the noise. My guess would be that the cats were behind it. I went to the kitchen to get a glass of water and discovered that Mom had started making stuffing. Remember, I said that Mom was going to do some kind of cooking or baking. I did not think it would be at 2:30 in the morning.

She honked for me at 3 to help her to the bathroom and I had to smile. She is going through the motions of calling me when she has to go to the bathroom, but will get up and cook in the middle of the night. She probably runs with scissors while I am not looking. I offered her a half of an Ambien, to see if it would help her and me get a little more shut eye. I was not able to go back to sleep, but enjoyed sitting at my computer and listening to Christmas music.

Mom was awake again at 5. I think all the stuffing she ate was backing up on her. I got her settled in bed and went to let Grace out and discovered that it was raining.

Thank you God, for this day so sweet, for best friends named Lynda, for the peace that comes with a shared prayer, for my hot pink Caddy fins and for the sense of comfort that comes in the early morning hours, before the rest of the world is awake. Love, Sue

DECEMBER 7, 2001

Yesterday was a very productive day for Mom. She also is having increasing problems with the pain in her left heel. She can hardly get around. If I don't hear back from the Podiatry Clinic this morning, I will be making some calls myself. Mom's mobility is critical in so many ways, but primarily her mood and her feeling independent.

Mom had decided that Thursday was going to be the day when she made her popcorn scramble, TV trash mix and her Mexican pick up sticks. Marilyn was going to come stay with Mom while I went to the store, but I did not feel like I could handle getting out. It had been raining and the humidity left me wiped out and working on each breath. Lynda had called and told me that she would run to the store and do whatever would help Mom and me. I was also pretty tired because I had been awake since about 2:30 a.m. It was not long before she came and picked up a check to be deposited, along with the grocery list. I imagined that she somehow knew that she and Mom were on this great mission to create wonderful Christmas memories and food.

We had some sandwiches when she returned from the store and visited for a while. I found myself getting really sleepy. I jumped at her suggestion that I lay down and take a nap, and she and Mom would hold down the fort. I even slept through the delivery of my liquid oxygen. I woke around 3:45 and was instantly aware of wonderful caramel smells coming from the kitchen. Lynda came and told me that when she told Mom that I was asleep that she said, "If she is sleeping, let's get busy, before she wakes up and starts staring at me!" Unfortunately, I still tend to stare when she is working in the kitchen. I am working on breaking myself of that habit. I was surprised to hear Mom tell Lynda and me that they were going to make all three recipes today. My response was,

"With what?" Lynda told me that Mom had proclaimed that they would just make do and improvise. Lynda began to gather the ingredients for the second recipe that they were going to make and the only ingredient on hand was butter. I laughed out loud. Lynda had assumed that she had a little more to work with than just butter. Mom was able to come up with a recipe using the cereal left from the popcorn scramble and added some fritos and seasonings and like magic they had created TV trash mix. Mom told Lynda that this really felt like Christmas to her. They were really stumped with the Mexican pick up sticks because they were left with only having butter on hand. Lynda ran to the store while the TV trash was cooking. Mom decided to lay down and rest while Lynda was gone. Lynda and Mom got the Mexican pick up sticks made.

Kelly surprised us with a visit. She gave me an early Christmas present. She gave me a toy hamster that sings and dances to *Kung Foo Fighting*. It had me rolling on the floor with laughter. I am glad that she knows me well enough to know how much fun I would have with it. We all enjoyed the evening. I told Mom that I should believe her when she says that she is going to do something.

Mom was having more and more trouble walking with this foot pain. She finally agreed to using the potty chair. Hopefully, this is only temporary. Once she gets this foot pain under control, she will be more mobile.

It was a 3-honk night.

Thank you God, for this day so sweet, for an afternoon nap, for the sounds and smell from Mom's kitchen, for Lynda's energy and enthusiasm and for a friend who knew that I could use a little hamster that knew the lyrics to *Kung Foo Fighting*. Love, Sue

DECEMBER 8, 2001

Yesterday had a frightening start to it. While I was finishing my morning note, Mom honked for me. Grace was laying in the doorway and I told her to hop up. When she went to stand up, she lost her balance and then her body went rigid for a few moments. She did not lose consciousness or bowel or bladder control, but she definitely had a small seizure. I made sure she was ok and went to help Mom. I was crying the whole time. I was afraid that she might have some increase in pressure in her head, because I found where she had thrown up and that goes hand in hand. While I was getting Mom situated, I called Lynda and asked her to please come quick because my Grace was sick. While I was getting ready, Grace appeared comfortable and did not seem to have trouble walking. I quickly put out a call to Diane and Becky to have them say a prayer. Mom called Bryant to see if he could come over. Right after Lynda arrived, Kathy, Mom's nurse, called and I busted out crying again. She offered words of comfort. I did not know, but Lynda called Kelly back to let her know about Grace and Kelly decided to leave work and drive across town, so I would not have to be alone if the news was bad.

They took Grace right in and gave her a thorough going over. I stood there struggling to hold back my tears. Grace has been by my side for thirteen and a half years. She has comforted me in so many ways, not to mention how she watches over Mom. She is also good for a laugh anytime. I swear she has a sense of humor. I told Dr. H. that I was losing my Mom and I knew that I could not stand to lose both of them at the same time. It was such a disorienting feeling. Deep down, I knew that if the problem was painful and she would suffer, that I would be there for her and would not fold when she needed me to keep a level head.

After Dr. H. finished examining her, he took time to explain what he thought was going on. Her eye exam did not show any signs of increased pressure in her brain. That was real good news, so the vomiting was a coincidence. Her heart, lungs, balance and blood work was fine. He explained that there are numerous reasons for a dog to have minor seizure activity, like she could have hopped up too quickly, and the change in her blood pressure might have triggered a little seizure. He also told me that it was very likely that she will never have another one. He did say that a seizure disorder was not necessarily a terminal event. We discussed what to do in the event of further seizures. He told me that I could relax, because Grace looked fine to him and she could go home. As I was walking out of the clinic, I looked up and Kelly drove up. I was shocked and started crying from relief. After Lynda called her, she told the folks at the office that there was an emergency and she had to leave. She had to have driven hard to make it to the clinic in that time. I hugged her and then I cried. Lynda and Kelly had gathered around, so Grace and I did not have to be alone. It did not surprise me that they were 100 percent there for me. I was just overwhelmed with gratitude for having such friends in my life.

Before I got home, I got a phone call from Lynda needing some information on Mom because Kathy was there. I was just a few minutes away, so Kathy would not have to wait long for the information she needed. When I got home, Kathy and Vicky were there. Everyone wanted to know about Grace, before we talked about Mom's medicine. Grace came in and greeted everyone and laid down in the middle of the floor and accepted all pats and hugs that were offered.

Kathy was very concerned about the increasing swelling in Mom's legs and thighs. She also was concerned about the increasing pain in her left foot. She was able to get in touch with the podiatry clinic and gave them Mom's insurance information. Mom agreed to start taking the lasix again and the Elavil at night. The Elavil might help with the burning pain that comes from the mass impacting clusters of nerves. In fact, the swelling is from the spread of the tumor in her pelvis.

After they left, I told Lynda that I was going to treat us to tacos in celebration of Grace's good report. While I was gone, Bryant came by and saw that the car was not there, so he went to the clinic assuming

I was still there. He came back to Mom's house, so he could find out about Grace. I was so touched that he came across town to see if he could help. While he was here, he cleaned out the fountain and spent some time visiting with Mom. I was still feeling shaky after the scare with Grace, so Lynda suggested that I lay down for a while. She had started a load of Mom's clothes and emptied the dishwasher. I did not take a nap, but I was able to rest and give my nerves a breather.

Janet arrived for a visit with Mom and me. Lynda and Janet were finally able to meet face to face. I had to show off the Christmas trees and my Santa collection. We all sat together in Mom's room and talked about the day and some funny stories that we had been giggling about. During our visit, Mom asked Lynda to slice up some tomatoes for her and fry a piece of Spam to go with it. We all know how irrational cravings can be.

Lynda had to leave after she had prepared Mom's snack. I gave her one last big hug and words of gratitude. Janet, Mom and I talked some about the different ways there are to come to God. It was soon time for Janet to leave. She had a Christmas party that she had to get ready for.

Mom and I spent some time talking about the day's activities. I watched her make these pretty bows out of wired ribbons. Mom is happiest when her hands are busy. I tucked Mom in and turned in early for the night.

It was a 2-honk night.

Thank you God, for this day so sweet, for the blessings that come with having Lynda and Kelly, not only as my friends, but my personal Angels, for Dr. H's words of comfort, for the visit with Janet and for the gift of Grace. Love, Sue

Mexican Pick-Up Sticks

2 3-ounce cans French Fried onions

1 7 ounce can potato sticks

1 package taco seasoning mix

2 cups Spanish peanuts

1/3 cup melted butter

    Combine onions, potato sticks and peanuts

    Place in a 9 X 13 baking dish

    Drizzle with melted butter and stir

    Sprinkle with taco seasoning

    Mix well

    Bake at 250° for 45 minutes stirring every 15 minutes

    Yields 2 quarts

DECEMBER 9, 2001

Mom had a better day yesterday. Her legs are beginning to look like legs, with the help of a lot of Lasix. She spent most of the day in bed with her legs propped up high. The only time she got out of bed, was to the bedside potty and to the kitchen to get her hair washed and styled. Becky came early, bringing all sorts of wonderful things. She had our groceries, Christmas gifts and a big batch of buttermilk fudge. We visited a little while then she put on her apron and got busy. I decided not to go out because there were things that I wanted to do in my room. Mom was kind of drowsy from the Elavil that she took the night before, so she tended to take small frequent naps. When she would wake, she would make more gold bows.

Becky found another big box of ornaments and I told her to put them back because I just did not have room on the tree. I have to decide which buildings of the North Pole Village I am going to put out. I would like to put it all out, but it would use up precious energy and time that I want to spend on other Christmas activities. I am running out of room for all my Santas. In spite of this, I feel like one can never have too many Santas. She also found the slimiest slug that she threatened me with. I was really scared that we would have a major incident. Baby sisters still revert back to old ways of scaring their older sister.

Uncle William called to tell us that Stephen had called to ask them to come to Denton. Uncle Dade was considered critical. He became tearful as he talked with Becky about this. All of our hearts and prayers go to the Spark's family. I called Diane and Bryant to let them know. Becky asked that I tell Mom. Mom would like to be there for her sister, but she isn't well enough to do this. I know that it is terrible to have someone so very sick and for it to be the holiday season on top of it. There should be a moratorium on sickness at Christmas. I remember when Dad was in the hospital at Christmas time and I could not understand how could everybody be celebrating when my Dad was so sick. As they say, life goes on. Right now all of our thoughts and prayers are in Denton with our beloved Uncle Dade, Aunt FiFi, Stephen and Susanne.

Becky finished working her magic, with a heavy dose of sweat and hard work on our home. She kissed us and headed home. Diane called to announce that she was able to walk for two hours and carry groceries and not get that tired feeling. She feels like the surgery was a great success. Mom asked me to put the navy bean soup on to cook. It soon filled the kitchen with wonderful smells. Navy beans and soup are two of her favorite foods. So navy bean soup is a big winner in Mom's eyes. I finished folding the clothes.

I have been watching Grace carefully. She has no interest in eating and has been very still. Still no seizure activity. Hopefully she will eat soon. Mom turned in early for the night.

It was a 1-honk night. When I let Grace out, I noticed that it was 32°. It was Rumba time. I excused Grace, because she was feeling under the weather. The cats were thankful that it was not square dance time.

Thank you God, for this day so sweet, for the gift of having an Uncle Dade in our lives, for Becky and her Saturday house makeovers, for Diane's two hour fatigue free walk, for navy bean soup and the return of cold weather. I am also asking for your prayers for Uncle Dade and his family. Love, Sue

DECEMBER 10, 2001

Mom had a quiet day yesterday. Her thoughts were in Denton with her sister and her family. Uncle William and Aunt MM went to Denton to see FiFi and Dade. Mom started her day watching church on TV. In an attempt to stay busy, Mom started reading the newspaper after the church services were over. We had a late brunch, which she seemed to enjoy. Grace finally ate some of her chicken today and I noticed a little spring in her step. Mom and I think she is on the road to recovery.

I watched out the window as our longtime neighbor had his estate sale. It is hard to believe that his home is sold and people are wandering through the house buying a lifetime of his belongings. We also received a call from our neighbor Pat, who told us that Gary, our next-door neighbor's, father died on Thanksgiving. Gary and Sue have experienced such losses. Sue's father died in October. Pat said that they did not want to bother us with their sad news. I wish that they would have let us know. Life goes on and neither Mom nor I are looking for any excuses to not be included in the happy or the sad.

I have decided not to put up my North Pole Village this year. I worried about not having Christmas with all of the trimmings. I think that sometimes the trimmings can interfere with the relaxing and peaceful part of the celebration. I am definitely in the Christmas spirit, but am aware of the need to pace myself. It would be easy for me to get all wound up in some of the trimmings and miss out on the quiet, intimate part of celebrating this last Christmas with my mother. She has told me that the house looks beautiful as it is now and she understands about how time consuming it is to get it all set up.

Bryant, Jacob and Sara came over and Bryant got the wheelchair out of the car for Mom. Mom hopped in the wheelchair and Sara pushed her all over the house to see what new decorations I had added. She wanted to listen to some Christmas music as she enjoyed looking at the tree. Several times she commented on how wonderful the house felt to her. She wanted to be rolled into the kitchen and have dinner at the table. She enjoyed being surrounded by her son and daughter and grandchildren. We talked about making a Rocky Road Cake for our friend Ralph's birthday. Mom is always on the lookout for reasons to cook for the people she loves. It was a school night, so Bryant and the kids needed to scoot home. Uncle William finally called. He said that Dade was not out of the woods and Stephen and Susanne had canceled their flights home. All of them are exhausted from staying at the hospital, but that is what you do when you have a loved one in ICU. I know that Aunt FiFi is comforted by their presence.

As usual Mom and I turned in early for the night.

Mom had a 4-honk night. She was restless and could not really relax. She was not hurting and for that I was thankful.

It was 32° when I let Grace out for her morning ritual. It was definitely twist and shout weather. Ringo panicked when he thought that the frost on the grass was snow. Max had to have him breathe into a brown paper sack to help him regain his composure.

Thank you God, for this day so sweet, for church services on TV, for Grace's bounce in her step, for the wheelchair ride that Sara gave Mom, for the excitement in making plans to bake a cake with Mom and for Bryant's help in moving our heavy plants to the patio. Please remember the Spark's family in your prayers. Love, Sue

DECEMBER 11, 2001

Sorry for the lateness of this note. This is going to be a very brief note. It has been chaotic here this morning. I also was trying to get ready to take Grace to be groomed. I hated leaving her. Mom had a quiet day yesterday. The highlight was when we made a Rocky Road Cake together. Uncle Dade continues to be in critical condition. Mom surprised me and slept through the night.

Thank you God, for this day so sweet, for Mom and I teaming up and making a cake and for a peaceful night's sleep. Love, Sue

DECEMBER 12, 2001

Yesterday was a nice day for Mom. Lynda came over to stay with Mom while I took Grace to be groomed and run a few errands. I really enjoy seeing how folks decorate their houses for Christmas. It was a rainy cold day and I cut my errand running short. When I returned home, I discovered that Lynda had been busy. Let me count the ways- trash gathered and taken to the alley, birds fed, cats fed and their litter box cleaned out, carpet vacuumed, dishwasher unloaded, my clothes folded, Mom entertained and she had made a wonderful tuna salad. It does not surprise me, but I feel so extraordinarily blessed to have a friend like Lynda, and to have her step in and automatically set our house right is something special and is important to me to acknowledge. Her attitude is, "What is the big deal? That is what friends do." She is right, but in this world where we all get so busy, it is a wonderful reminder that there are people that remember the old ways. I feel like Lynda and Marilyn, at times, have been involved in all-day barn raisings and bringing in the crops.

Uncle William, Aunt MM and Lee came by to see Mom. Our conversation centered on our family in Denton and how we hoped that they were comforted with all our thoughts and prayers that we were sending their way. After they left for home Lynda helped Mom make another Rocky Road Cake for Gary and Sue. While we were waiting for it to bake, we all played a game of Skip-Bo. Lynda won the game and whupped us soundly. I begin to feel like I was coming down with something. I found myself putting on a sweater. I had trouble deciding if I was hot or cold. I think I was probably running a temperature. Mom decided to lay down and take a nap and Lynda had volunteered to go pick up Grace from the groomer. I was missing her terribly. In fact, I dreaded coming home to an empty house after I had left her at the groomer. She really did need to be shed. Her rear end looked like she was wearing a thatched roof.

Kelly called and offered words of comfort. She also had trouble leaving her pup at the groomer. I found myself keeping vigil at my window. The weather had even gotten worse and I knew that they had probably got caught in it. Lynda and Grace arrived and Mom and I were all over her. One would have thought that she had been on a long trip. Before Lynda left, we talked about me going to the doctor on Wednesday. I can't afford to have anything impact my ability to care for Mom.

Mom and I both turned in early for the night. It was a 3-honk night. Mom has problems with her mouth becoming painfully dry. She has promised that she won't try to get up on her own, so when her mouth gets dry, she honks for me.

Thank you God, for this day so sweet, for the warm feelings from seeing all the Christmas decorations on all the houses, for Grace's smooth new look, for the special blessings of friends that come and help raise barns and bring in the crops, for the comfort of being in a family that comes to you in prayer. Please remember our family in Denton in your prayers today. Love, Sue

DECEMBER 13, 2001

Yesterday was basically ok for Mom, but she was troubled with anxiety for a portion of the day. The last several days, she has complained of nightmares where she has died. She told me yesterday that she was afraid that she was dying. I asked her what symptoms she was having that would contribute to the feeling that she was dying. All she could come up with was a dry mouth. Also when she first woke up, she did not feel like she could move. I had her wiggle her toes and move her legs. She was able to stand and transfer into the wheelchair. I told her that she was not crazy. I explained that fears based on unreal experiences had the same powers that came from fears based on a real threat. After Vicky helped Mom get cleaned up, Mom asked for some medication to help calm down some of her anxiety. She understood that the pill would probably make her sleepy. I helped her back to bed and started getting dressed, so I would make it to my doctor's appointment on time. Lynda came to watch over Mom while I was gone.

The doctor told me that I probably had a virus or the beginning of the flu. I had been running a temperature and feeling kind of punk. The good news was that my lungs were clear. He gave me a couple of prescriptions and told me to take it easy. I called to check on Mom and Lynda told me that she had been asleep since I had been gone. When I got home and opened the front door, I was met with wonderful smells from the kitchen. Lynda had prepared pork chops and potatoes with onions. Gracie was crying and hooting, as she greeted me and her enthusiastic greeting woke Mom from her sleep. Mom seemed relieved when I told her that I would be like new in a couple of days. She reported that her anxiety was gone.

Lynda needed to head on home, so we hugged and said our good byes. Mom decided to get up and come to the kitchen table for dinner. She talked again about how scared she was last night. She did respond to my suggestions that she tell herself that she was safe at this time and I was only a step away if she needed me.

We both turned in early, as this has become a routine for us. Mom honked for me around 1:15. She was telling me that something was wrong and she could not move. She was able to wiggle her toes and move her legs. When it was time for her to transfer she was a little shaky. I was able to get her in the bathroom and with a little help from me she was able to sit on the toilet. She asked that I call Bryant, because she was sure that it would be impossible for her to stand up. I put on my psychiatric nursing cap and decided that I was seeing a panic attack. Mom is weak, but there is no reason that she can't move. In fact, earlier she had walked to the kitchen, living room and her bedroom with the use of her walker. I was eventually able to convince her that I could provide all the help she would need. Mom was able to transfer to the bed with some assistance from me.

She did not honk the rest of the night, but I was up checking on her. I think in the back of my mind, I had an irrational fear that maybe her fear was based on some real experience that was hidden from me.

Thank you God, for this day so sweet, for Mom talking with me about her concerns and fears, for wonderful pan-fried potatoes and onions, for the medication that will ease my symptoms and for the excitement of receiving Christmas cards from old friends. Uncle Dade seems to be a little more stable. Thank you for all your prayers. He is not out of the woods, so your continued prayers would be appreciated. Love, Sue

DECEMBER 14, 2001

Mom had a difficult day yesterday. After I finished writing my morning note, I decided to go check on Mom. Becky was on the phone at the time and I did not want to hang up until I had checked to see if Mom was ok. She has been sleeping with her eyes half open and it shocks me when I first look at her. Mom was awake when I checked on her. She told me that she could not move and she was sure that she was dying. I was not expecting to hear her make such a statement. I did ask her what made her feel like she was dying. She told me that she felt like her very life force had drained out of her. I attempted to explain that Lasix could make her feel that way. While talking to her, I noticed that her eyes and the hollows of her cheeks had a sunken in look. It looked like those children that you see on TV that are starving. I imagine that we had overdone on the Lasix. Whatever swelling that was left was probably lymphedema. Lasix won't take that away. Mom resisted all explanations I had to offer. She also was not responding to my attempts to comfort her. I told her that I was going to call Kathy. I felt like Kathy might have a different type of ability to convince her that she was weak from the lasix, but she was stable.

Mom asked to get in the wheelchair and sit in the living room. I sat down next to her. She turned to me and said, "Sue, please pray with me." Her prayer was one that you might hear someone pray prior to their death. She asked for forgiveness of her many sins. She also prayed that God continue to watch and care for her children. I had tears in my eyes by this time. After her prayer, she turned to me and told me how truly thankful she was to have had me take such good care of her. It was important that all of her children know how much they were loved and how special and unique she thought we all were.

I tried one more time to comfort Mom. I told her that if I thought she was dying or Kathy told me that she was dying, I would never keep it a secret from her. This was her life and she had the absolute right to know if there was concern that death was close. I also reassured her that I would call all her children to be at her side when the time arrived. I told her that her vital signs were stable and there were none of the physical signs one sees when death is near. She just patted my hand, gave me a knowing look and told me that she loved me.

Kathy soon arrived and basically told Mom the same things I had told her. Kathy finally told her that she had a lot more baking that needed to be done and not just for Christmas. I told her that New Year's was around the corner and there was cornbread, black-eyed peas and cabbage to prepare. Kathy nodded her head in agreement.

Mom did smile and said, "If that is what you think, Suzie and I have some fruitcake cookies to bake, not to mention the gingerbread house." Mom agreed to try to drink a lot of juice and water to rehydrate herself. I did have some nagging concerning Mom telling us what we wanted to hear. She fell asleep soon after Kathy left.

I woke her a little later and sat with her while she sipped on some V8 juice. She told me that she still felt lifeless, but if we said she wasn't dying, she guessed she would have to take our word. I was not real convinced by her speech or her effect that she had accepted our explanations. Mom drank about six ounces of juice then fell asleep again. I checked on her frequently because I thought she might be playing possum. I was afraid that she would pretend sleep to avoid talking. I wish I was a mind reader and could tell if there were other things that were frightening her that she had not told me. She slept for most of the day. A few times I was able to get her to drink some water and eat some chipped ice, which has become a favorite.

At dinner time I woke her and insisted that she try to drink some broth from the navy bean soup and a small cup of Jell-O. She drank maybe four ounces of soup and ate half of her Jell-O cup. I decided to take a firm approach about her taking her Zoloft and Synthroid. She was not happy, but she took it. Bryant and Jacob surprised us with a short visit. Mother started looking agitated. Bryant left to go get dinner for Jacob and was coming right back. I went in Mom's room and offered her a glass of water to take her pain pill with. She made a face and waved me off. I had just recently filled her glass with fresh water, but I filled her glass again. When I took the water to Mom, she motioned for me to lean down so she could whisper in my ear. Mom expressed a fear that Bryant was going to kill her because he had told her in the past that she must not die before him. To say that I was shocked is an understatement. She was afraid that he had poisoned her water. From my experience as a psychiatric nurse, all I could do was tell her she was safe and I would not let anyone harm her. I knew that I could not use rational thought to fight against her irrational fears.

After he left, I told Mom that I had locked the front door and that she was safe. Well, she got agitated and wanted the front door unlocked so Bryant could get in to help her if she was choking and help her stay alive. She told me that she knew that I would not let him in if he knocked. I went and pretended that I was unlocking the door. I could only hope that she would not become paranoid about me. I think all of this irrational thinking is coming from her being dehydrated. I tucked her in and said good night.

Mom did not honk for me last night. I was up frequently checking on her. She was awake at 3:30 and I asked her if she wanted some ice. She whispered that she was unable to move. This is the third morning in a row that she has expressed that fear. I fed her some ice and she did use her hands to pick up some ice that fell on her chest. My guess would be that Mom still has some delusions in place. It is times like this when I look around to see if there is a grown up in the room to take over.

Thank you God, for this day so sweet, for Becky's comforting morning phone call, for Kathy making time in her day to make an extra visit to see Mom, for Mom's request that I hear her prayer, for all my education that is helping me to care for and have an understanding of Mom's fears and for the comfort I feel when I listen to Willie Nelson's CD *How Great Thou Art*. Uncle Dade is still in ICU. I so appreciate your prayers for his family. Love, Sue

Fruit Cake Cookies

1/4 cup butter

1 pound mixed fruit cake fruit or ½ pound each candied pineapple and cherries

1 pound white raisins

½ cup flour (for flouring fruit)

1 pound pecans

dough

½ cup brown sugar

2 eggs

1 cup flour

1/3 cup orange pineapple juice

1 tsp

soda dissolved in 1½ Tbs sweet milk

dash salt

½ tsp allspice

½ tsp cloves

1 tsp cinnamon

    Cut fruit and toss with flour

    Mix dough

    Pour batter over fruit, this is just enough batter to stick fruit together

    Drop by teaspoon on a greased cookie sheet

    Top each cookie with a piece of cherry

    Bake at 350° for 15 minutes

    Yields 85-100 cookies

DECEMBER 16, 2001—FROM DIANE

I just talked to Sue. Hospice is going to start continuous care and they say that it could be in the next twenty four hours. I am going to try to pull things together so that I can leave tomorrow morning.   ~ Diane

DECEMBER 16, 2001

Yesterday was the most difficult day that Mom and her children have faced. Mom has taken a dramatic turn for the worse. I guess I should have listened to Mom more closely when she kept telling me that she was dying. I thought I was looking at someone that was dehydrated and this could be corrected with increasing fluid and food intake. I fixed a fried egg in a hole and some sausage for breakfast. I also had frozen some juice that I shaved, kind of like a snow cone. It took forever for Mom to finish her breakfast. I was not feeling ok with this stern nurse role I found myself in. I felt like I had been getting mixed signals from Mom. She had told me the day before that she did not want to die. Saturday her behavior was saying something very different. Mom was sitting in the recliner when Becky arrived with all the groceries, Christ-

mas presents and all of her homemade goodies. While Becky was freshening the house, I went to pick up a couple of movies and some soup from Schlotzky's. We wheeled Mom into the kitchen to eat her soup. It was painful watching her look at the soup with such dread. I knew I was needing to hear her tell me what she

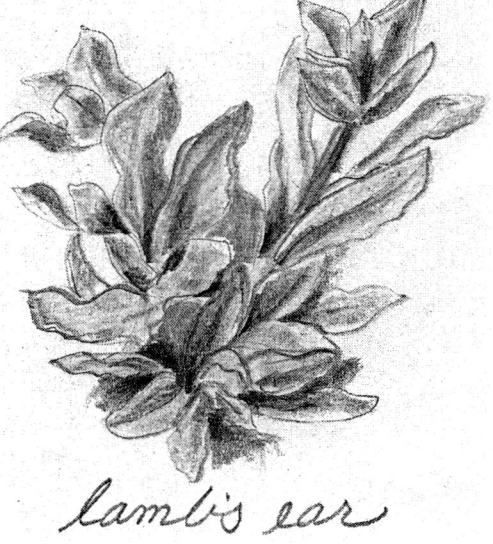

lamb's ear

really wanted us to do. I asked Mom if she was giving up and letting go. She told Becky and me that she was ready to die, that she was so weary and could no longer struggle with eating or drinking. I watched as Becky broke into tears. It was the first time since Mom got sick that I had seen her cry.

Mom reached over, caressed her head and told her that she loved her and knew this was difficult for us to hear. We asked Mom if she did not feel like she could hold on till next Friday when Debi and Jenny would be able to say their good byes. She said that she was sorry, but she did not think she could hold on. I told Mom that I did not want her last memories of me to be of me badgering her to eat and drink. I wanted her to remember my soft touches, the bedtime prayers, goodnight kisses, how many times I had told her that I loved her and feeding her shaved ice in the middle of the night when she complained of a dry mouth. I told Mom that it would be hard, but I would respect her wishes. Becky and I cried as we talked about how much she would be missed. We told her that she needed to know that we knew how to take care of ourselves and would make her proud of us. I decided to have her open one of her Christmas presents from me. It was a pink chenille bed jacket. I told her that everyone would be wanting to pet her because it was so soft. She smiled and told me to go get Becky's present from the living room. Becky broke into tears when she saw Aunt Lois's biscuit jar. She hugged Mom and went to her car to retrieve a present that Mom had picked out for me. I became tearful when I saw that it was a special frame that would hold a paw print and a picture of Grace. Mom asked me to call Diane and Bryant. Becky helped me get Mom back in bed and she kissed her good bye. I told Becky that I would be ok and she needed to head home.

It was not long before Bryant had arrived. He had brought this Santa doll that he had carved out of clay at Mom's direction. He had even made the body. It was beautiful and there were more tears shed.

Bryant fed Mom some shaved ice. I went to check her pulse and was concerned that it had dropped to 60. Bryant and I talked and decided to call hospice. They have a continuous care plan for people that are nearing death. They provide round the clock care. Lisa, the on-call nurse, said that it might take a while, but she would come and check on Mom. The weather has been miserable with all of the heavy rain.

Lisa arrived around 11:00 p.m. She also felt that Mom was failing. She was not responsive at times and her pulse had dropped to 48. Lisa felt that Mom qualified for continuous care, but there was no available staff to come right away. She hoped that by morning she would have somebody that could stay with Mom around the clock. She also called in a prescription for liquid Oxycontin. I was relieved because I did not know how we were going to give her pain medicine. I told Bryant and Lisa, that they could leave. I was really wanting the house to myself. I planned on checking on Mom every hour and a half to two hours. They left and I kissed Mom good night.

I went to call Diane and told her that it was time for her to come. We shared some tears over the phone. I laid down, but I kept hearing my name called. The pharmacy delivered the medicine about 2 a.m. Each time that I checked on her, I offered her some shaved ice. Becky checked in around 7 a.m. to see how the night went and Diane called a few moments later.

Thank you God, for this day so sweet, for a mother's honesty, for early Christmas presents, for hugs from my mother, sister and brother and for the comfort of prayer. Love, Sue

DECEMBER 17, 2001
Linc is an old friend of Sally's

Yesterday was a long day for all concerned. Mom is actively dying now. Hospice is trying to find nursing staff to come and take care of Mom. I called Lynda and Kelly early Saturday morning to tell them about the changes in Mom. They came right over. Lynda helped me with turning and helping her get comfortable. There were many tears being shed. Lynda squared her shoulders and asked what needed to be done. I wanted to be able to lay down for about thirty minutes. I told her that the kitchen table was covered with packages from her to her children and friends. Lynda and Kelly wrapped every last package in this house. They used all sorts of pretty ribbons and bows. While they were wrapping Janet came by to offer prayer and support. Marilyn came by to say her good byes. Pat came by with banana bread and fruitcake. There were phone calls from old friends. I had also called Linc to tell him about Mom. I wanted him to be able to say good bye. Vicky, Mom's aide, came by to say good bye. I felt so disoriented.

Lisa called to let us know that Mabel would be Mom's nurse from 7 p.m. to 7 a.m. Marilyn stayed for a while. She has been right there for Mom all the way. She told me that she would let Carol know about Mom. While Janet was here, she made some phone calls to some motels that we thought offered free rooms for family that was coming from out of town. Comfort Inn at 635 and Northwest Highway offered a free room for five days. There are really nice people out there. Tom had read the article about the participating motels that offered this kind of service and told us that it would be worth checking into. It was surely welcomed information.

Diane, Gordon and Jenny were on their way to Dallas. They were going to have to drive through driving rain for most of the trip. The important thing was they were coming. Aunt FiFi called and was tearful. Uncle Dade is also failing. She is faced with losing her baby sister and her husband. Becky, Tom and Sherri arrived around 4:30. Sherri was struggling with tears like all of us were. Tom checked on Mom and then set out to do some important repair work on the house. Becky helped to straighten out Mom's room and put up the rest of the wrapping papers in the attic. Diane, Gordon and Jenny arrived around

8 p.m. I hugged them all and told them that I had to lay down, before I fell down. I vaguely remember Lisa, the nurse, talking to me. I slept straight through the night.

When I woke, I found Michele, the day nurse, in Mom's room with Mabel, the night shift nurse. Mabel told me that Mom had a fairly restful night. She had medicated her for pain several times and turned her and had given her a bath. Mom had been well-taken care of during the night. Michele had observed that Mom's knees were beginning to mottle which is one of the signs of impending death. Her vital signs are stable right now. I woke Diane to tell her of the changes in Mom.

Thank you God, for this day so sweet, for Lynda and Kelly, I would not have made it through the day without them, for Janet's prayers, for all the friends and family that have gathered close by, for seeing Diane, Gordon and Jenny safely to our home, for your promise to walk with us during this final journey and your preparing a place for my Mother to come and rest. Love, Sue

DECEMBER 18, 2001

Yesterday was another day full of tears and good byes. Mom's fingers began to darken and her nurse told us that it might be a good idea to call the family that was not there. I called Becky and Uncle William. Bryant left to get Jacob and Sara so they could say their good byes. Jenny sat at Mom's side and held her hand for the longest time. We all gathered and told Mom that we were here and we knew that she was tired and ready to let go. We spoke of how her mother, father, brother and her husband were waiting for her. Mom did tell Jenny that she was going to have to let her go. We have CD's of all of Mom's favorite hymns playing continuously in the background. It is very soothing to us and I can only hope is soothing to Mom. Jacob and Sara were very tearful when they leaned down to kiss Mom good bye. Mom was their special Granny that could work magic. Becky, Tom and Sherri arrived and went right to Mom's bedside. Uncle William, Aunt MM and Lee arrived and also went to Mom's bedside. We all thought that death was just moments away. Mom surprised us with having a stable pulse. I guess no one really knows exactly when the moment of death will arrive. Margaret was able to come by and say her good byes. Lisa also came by with Dria and Grace wearing the snowmen shirts that Mom had given them for Christmas. Mom opened her eyes and smiled at them.

All Mom's children gathered to talk about making the funeral arrangements for Mom. It was decided that Diane and I would go and begin the process. We had decided to have Sparkman Hillcrest as the funeral home. All of the details in planning a funeral are simply overwhelming. They had agreed to allow us to sit up through the night with Mom's body at the funeral home. I had done that with Dad and want to do the same thing with Mom. After we finished there, we had to run by the store and pick up some coffee and milk. We did not get home till a little after 6. Becky told us that Aunt FiFi and Stephen had come from Dade's bedside to Mom's bedside. Susanne had insisted that her mother come and say good bye to her sister. Aunt FiFi had told Becky that they were going to remove Uncle Dade's ventilator Tuesday morning. My heart goes out to all of them. It is a lot to bear, losing your husband and your sister at the same time. While we were gone, Becky took out trash, did three loads of wash, made four pots of coffee and vacuumed. She responds to stress with a need to create order. I am sure glad we all approach things in a different way. Mom always said that her children were all so different and complimented each other with their talents. As a group we could handle anything. She is right, we are pulling together and doing what we do the best.

During the day Mom's nurse, Kathy, came along with Marion, the social worker. Later in the evening Janet, the chaplain for hospice, came by to offer support. Diane and I were at the numb stage. Joe, Lisa's husband, also came by in the evening to say his good byes. He was pleased when I asked him if he would be one of Mom's pallbearers. It was 8 p.m. before we ate.

Before I went to bed I went and said our evening prayers, including Now I Lay Me Down to Sleep. We told Mabel, the nurse, to let us know if there were any changes in the night. She woke us around 1 or 1:30, to tell us that Mom's fingertips had darkened considerably. Her pulse was still stable. We sat with Mom for a while then returned to bed. I got up at 6 and went and sat with Mom for a while. She did not open her eyes, but she knew I was there. She would nod her head when I spoke to her.

Thank you God, for this day so sweet, for the tender nursing care Mom is receiving, for how our family is coming together at this time, for Aunt FiFi and Stephen having a chance to say good bye to Mom, for Dria and Grace and their snowmen shirts and for the peace, support and comfort that your promises bring to our hearts. Love, Sue

DECEMBER 19, 2001
Debi is Becky's daughter

Mom's vital signs were more stable yesterday. There continue to be good byes that were made through the day and evening. Marilyn called and wanted to know if there was anything she could do. Before we knew it, Marilyn had arrived with a thirty cup coffee urn, a huge ham, cheesecake, croissants, crackers and spinach dip. Uncle William and Aunt MM spent some time with Mom this morning. Marilyn had a chance to finally meet them. Bryant was also here several times during the day. He sat with Mom and he would feed her shaved ice. Diane and I needed to go and finish the funeral arrangements at Sparkman Hillcrest. I did not want to leave Jenny alone with the nurse and Mom. Bryant had to leave and could come back later to stay with Mom, but Diane and I needed to finish up with the funeral arrangements.

Marilyn offered to stay with Jenny while we were gone. Here is another example of how blessed Mom and this family are to have friends that will help you bring in the crops.

I had my cell phone and we left to tie up as many loose ends as possible. At times, Diane and I would reach out and just hold hands. Words were not needed at those times. At Sparkman's I did shed a few tears when we were looking at the memorial book and trying to decide on the style and content of the service folders. I had held myself together the day before at Sparkman's. I don't know what there was about the memorial book and the service folders that brought on the tears. I am not doing a lot of holding back on the tears. I figure that I don't have anything to prove to anybody. This is one of the saddest times in, not just my life, but all of her family and friends.

Mom was such a wonderful example of a woman who lived as an example to others. She would not see her self that way. She was a teacher in the truest since of the word. She taught us about unconditional love, the importance of family, there was reward in hard work and a job well done, how valuable the phone numbers, addresses and a list of birthdays and other celebrations were, in staying in touch with family and friends, how the easy way was not always the best way. She showed me that hard work, patience, dirty hands and a good system for watering could create a breathtaking perennial and annual garden, full of spectacular butterflies and every kind of bird imaginable. And the excitement that comes with stumbling onto a good garage or estate sale, how she loved Grace Elizabeth and would remember her birthday, how clipping coupons does help with the grocery budget, how there was always room for one more plate at the table, how a well stocked pantry and refrigerator/freezer could be a blessing, how to cook really good beans, meatloaf with red sauce, chicken and dumplings, corn pudding, chalupas and all of her cakes and pies. The last thing Mom baked was a Rocky Road cake on Wednesday for Gary and Sue next door. And how important it is to write your thank you notes, how it is easier to see the good, rather than the bad, in an experience, how enjoyable a game of scrabble with Diane is, as well as a game of Skip-Bo with her family and friends can be, how healing a heartfelt apology is, how it is just as easy, as well as important, to have good handwriting, how doing your homework really pays off, how wonderful it is to receive a really good back scratching, how a really deep laugh can clear your head, how a little imagination, glue and paint can transform a plain, little girl's room into something magical, how fortunate we were that our Mom made our school clothes, how wonderful it is to have a linen closet full of old linens. And how warm a home feels when you have pictures and photographs on the wall. And what a difference it made in children's lives to grow up going to Sunday school and church and how faith and prayer can see you through your darkest hour. There is not a part of my life that has not been molded by my mother's loving hands and heart. I also know that is true of all of the other people that were a part of my Mother's life.

Jenny helped me to prepare dinner. I showed her how to make green chili rice. Marilyn's wonderful ham completed dinner. Our neighbors, Pat and Sue, came over to say their good byes to Mom.

Mom had a peaceful day. She is still able to acknowledge when we are in the room. She seldom opens her eyes, but will respond yes or no and often give us a smile. Diane and I went in to say good night to Mom. I said our nightly prayers like we had been doing every night for a long time. Diane had folded herself up on the love seat and had fallen asleep. She was awake around 4 a.m. and Grace also wanted to go out. I did not want to go back to sleep, so I sat up with Mom for a while. She does look peaceful as she sleeps. Becky called early to tell us that Debi had arrived from New York and they would be here around 1 p.m.

Thank you God, for this day so sweet, for the comfort that Marilyn gave us, for the wonderful memories I have of my Mother, for Jenny's help in the kitchen, for the knowledge that Mom is receiving the most excellent and tender nursing care, for reaching out and finding Diane's hand, for the quiet conversations with Becky and Bryant and for how richly you blessed us when you chose Altha "Sally" Warenskjold Tittle as our mother and teacher. Love, Sue

DECEMBER 20, 2001

Mother had a peaceful day yesterday. She was more alert and responsive. It seems like she might be rallying one last time. We know that her status could literally change in a heartbeat. I sat with Mom for a while, before the rest of the house woke up. It is so peaceful in her room. There are beautiful flowers from Marilyn on her bedside table, hand painted pictures from Sara and Jacob, Christmas sheets on the bed, a beautiful Christmas quilt covering her. She is wearing some Angel pajamas that Becky had given her, comforting hymns playing in the background, a magical 3-foot Christmas tree on her chest of drawers at the end of her bed along with Christmas cards from friends. Grace is in often checking on her Granny, and her children and grandchildren have all gathered around to be with her as she makes her journey home.

Linc came to say his good byes. He was surprised at how emotional he became. Diane and I hugged him and told him it was good that he came to see Mom. Kathy, Mom's nurse, came by to check on Mom. I had a very animated conversation with her about the changes that hospice was trying to make in Mom's nursing care. They were wanting to pull Mom's wonderful nurses to another case in Fort Worth. Michele, Mom's day nurse, was also upset. I was very plain spoken about how I did understand about trying to arrange coverage for all the on-going cases...BUT that was not my problem. My goal was to make sure that my mom got the best nursing care available and a big part of good care is continuity of care. I told all involved that not only could I make a racket, but I had a sister named Becky that they did not want to meet. For right now, it seems like we have the nursing coverage straightened out.

Uncle William and Aunt MM came for their daily visit. They had not been gone long when Becky, Sherri and Debi arrived. Debi took an earlier flight from New York, so she could see her Granny. While Becky was here, Diane and I went to McShann's Florist and chose the casket spray. While we were gone, Becky did her magic in the house. After Becky and her girls left, I went to the grocery store for more apple juice. Mom has really increased her fluid intake. She is craving shaved ice and frozen fruit juices that have also been transformed by Mom's shaved ice machine. That ice shaver is one of the best investments I have made.

We had dinner when I returned from the store. I thought Mom would enjoy listening to *Wheel of Fortune*. It is one of her favorite game shows. She asked for her glasses and that is when the panic set in my heart. We could not find her glasses. I have a horrible habit of gathering up glasses that are laying around. I have all of Mom's old eyeglasses from ten and fifteen years ago. I also have some of Becky's old glasses. I even have several pairs of Lynda's glasses. The steroids had really played a number on my eyesight, so I have been continually searching for the perfect pair of glasses. Mind you, I have my own prescription for glasses. Any way, I was frantic and came and told Diane that I had lost Mom's glasses. She tried to maintain composure, but it did not last. She laughed so hard that she slid out of her chair on the floor. I found in my basket an older pair of Mom's glasses and I put them on her so she could watch *Wheel of Fortune*. Diane helped me look, but I have glasses in every room of the house. She tried to get me to see the humor in all of this, but initially it was hard. Even Mom was very vocal in telling me not to worry that they would show up. In the meantime, Mabel, Mom's 7 p.m. to 7 a.m. nurse, arrived and identified a pair of glasses as Mother's. I was of the opinion that they were an old pair that belonged to Bryant. Aunt FiFi called and I confessed my sins and she laughed and also told me that it was going to be ok.

It had been a long day for her. Uncle Dade is still in ICU and is continuing to decline. Later, when I was in Mom's room, Mabel asked Mom if she wanted to take off her glasses. Mom smiled and said, "No thank you." I guess she wasn't letting go of the pair of glasses she had on-at least while I was around. I told Diane how Mom had declined taking off her glasses and she again laughed so hard that she slid off of the love seat. I am warning anybody that comes over to the house to not take their glasses off—at least while I am in the room.

Bryant, Jacob and Sara came by for a visit. Jacob had painted a wonderful picture for Mom. Mom had a big grin on her face as she heard how they are excelling in school. Even though Mom was sleeping, I went on and said our prayers, like we had been doing all along. When I went to check on Mom early this morning, I discovered Gordon crunched up on the love seat with Mom's laundry covering him. He had sheets, towels and pajamas piled all over him. For a moment, I thought about waking Diane, but I decided to ignore the sitting room and go and check on Mom. Mabel told me that Mom had a restful night. Mom was awake and smiled when she saw me. I noticed how her fingertips had begun to darken again. All of her vital signs are strong and stable. The poor circulation in the fingertips is a sign of Mom's circulatory system being compromised. I held her hands to try to warm them.

Thank you God, for this day so sweet, for the quiet time spent with my Mom, for Debi being able to come and see her Granny, for Linc's visit, for the phone calls and the emails from friends, for having a sister like Becky that would make hospice think twice about changing things, for the smile on Mom's face after hearing about Jacob and Sara's good grades, for Diane's laughter, for Mom's words of comfort to me about her glasses, for Mom's nurses and for a peaceful night's sleep. Love, Sue

DECEMBER 21, 2001

Yesterday was difficult. Mom was alert and responsive early in the day. She was really craving frozen shaved apple juice, which she calls yellow ice. As the day progressed, Mom's pain and restlessness increased. Janet and Kathy arrived around the same time. While we were around the bed Mom said loudly, "Please let me die." All of us were quick to assure her that we were trying to get the pain under control, not prolong her time. Diane and I, once again, told Mom that we loved her enough to let her go and that she had taught us well how to take care of ourselves. We told her that her mother, father, husband and brother were all waiting for her. All I wanted for Mom was to get her easy. Kathy worked hard trying to get the orders from the doctor for changes in her medication. Kathy told us that we were probably seeing something called terminal restlessness. It is one of the last stages of the dying process. Janet offered to take Jenny to the store to get some smokes, diet Dr. Pepper and bread. This was certainly a blessing. I did not want to leave Mom, and Diane's back was really bothering her. They have a topical cream that helps to calm and sedate. We were told that the pharmacy would deliver as soon as possible. Kathy and Janet had lots of hugs and soft comforting words for us all. This was an example of hospice at its best.

We were also agitated because Mother's night nurse was not going to be Mabel. She had dental work and was not able to come last night. Lisa and Dria came over to see Mom and also see if there was anything else that she could do. Earlier she had sent over platters of food. It was a welcome break to see Dria smile and point to all the ornaments on the Christmas tree. After they left, Janice, the agency night nurse arrived. When she first arrived it looked like she was setting up a picnic. I was sitting by Mom's side and she said very loudly, "Looky at her thumb!" Mom's fingertips were very dusky. Diane and I knew that we would be up all night. Jenny had gotten tearful and feeling helpless. We all talked about how hard it was to simply wait. When I laid down, we were still waiting for her medicine to be delivered. Diane was going to wake me around 1 a.m.

I got up a little after midnight and found Diane still trying to track what happened to Mom's pain medicine. Evidently hospice and the pharmacy dropped the ball. They had to have a pharmacy in Fort Worth prepare and deliver Mom's pain medicine. It was close to 3 a.m. before it was delivered. This has been the worst time for Mom and us. She seemed to calm a little after she had the topical cream applied. It was hard to hear Mom's hymns for all the smacking noises that this nurse was making. I started to count the hours till Michele would return to care for Mom. Diane was in the kitchen with me when I went to get the baggy with Grace's turkey and found that it was gone. I call it her spa diet. She has turkey or chicken every morning. Well, the night nurse ate Grace's turkey. I did not think that I had to hide my dog's food. This nurse won't be returning tonight. Once was way too much.

Michele finally arrived and began to set things right. I am typing this note at 8:30 a.m. and Mom's blood pressure is dropping and her heart rate and respiration's are increasing. It probably won't be much longer. I am ready to let Mom go.

Thank you God, for this day so sweet, for yellow ice, for the opportunity to tell Mom that we did not want her to stay one moment longer than God intended and how much we loved her, for good neighbors, for the care that Kathy and Janet gave us, for Michele's tender care of Mom, for the stamina to stay awake and watch over Mom, for Jenny's maximum service and for a clear, cold, first day of winter. Love, Sue

DECEMBER 22, 2001

Mother had a peaceful day yesterday. Her blood pressure was low, but I think Mom's heart is so strong that it has been able to compensate for the fluctuations in her blood pressure. We thought she was hours if not moments away from death. Her fingers and feet had darkened again. She was not able to take any of the shaved ice we would offer her. My Uncle William and Aunt MM stayed with us for most of the morning. Uncle William did leave to go get one of Mom's prescriptions, so she would not have to wait. Aunt MM kept herself busy making sandwiches and coffee. Our Aunt FiFi called to update us on Uncle Dade. They had planned to take him off of life support on Saturday, but one of the doctor's had suggested they try one other type of medical intervention, before taking that final step. What a terrible position that they are in, trying to figure out the best care for Uncle Dade.

Becky called frequently through the day. She felt like she had made her good byes and felt like she needed to keep busy. Bryant, Jacob and

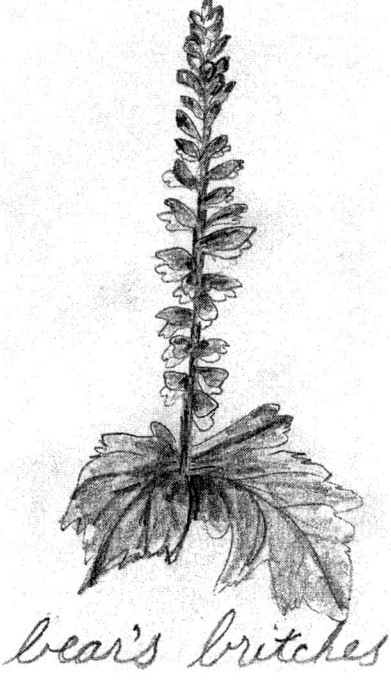

bear's britches

Sara came over and sat and talked to Mom. Bryant certainly has his hands full trying to make sure that their Santa Claus is all taken care of, in between being with Mom and getting a little sleep. Cil and Delbert came to our rescue when Delbert brought more chicken thighs for us to cook for our night nurse, Grace Elizabeth. He also brought some of Cil's wonderful homemade fudge and banana bread. Mom and I could not have been any more richly blessed with the wonderful friends that surround us.

Billy also arrived from Beaumont. He is Jenny's boyfriend and is spending Christmas with us. He had only been here for a short time, before he started taking out the trash and helping to run errands. He is an absolutely delightful young man and I am so glad he is here with us. After he got things squared away in the house, he went to register for the room at the Comfort Inn on Northwest Highway. Comfort Inn donates rooms to family coming from out of town to visit families that are in hospice or are here for a funeral. It truly is a wonderful service that they provide. Kathy came to check on Mom's status and ended up staying a while. We all got to telling about different funny times we had all experienced. The house was full of all our laughter. It felt so good to let go and laugh like we did in Mom's kitchen. As the night progressed, Mom appeared more responsive and was letting us know that she wanted some ice. Her fingers even began to pink up again. Kathy and I talked about how we had never seen someone alternate between apparent circulatory failure and then for it to appear that it had reversed itself. Of course, Mom has always defied the odds.

We were so glad when we saw Mabel come at 7 p.m. Diane and I both knew that we would probably be able to get some rest with her here. I went in and said my prayers with Mom around 8 p.m. Mabel told me that she would wake me if there were any changes in Mom. I don't remember my head hitting the pillow. Diane stayed with Mom until 10 p.m. and then Bryant came and sat with Mom until midnight. When I went to check on Mom at 6 a.m. Mabel told me that she had a very restful night. I noticed that Mom's fingers had pinked up. Michele, Mom's day nurse, arrived at 7 a.m. This will be her last shift with Mom. We will really miss her tender care of Mom.

Thank you God, for this day so sweet, for Mom's peaceful day and night, for Cil and Delbert replacing the night nurse's chicken, for the comfort of having Uncle William and Aunt MM with us, for Billy's safe trip to Dallas, for the generosity of the Comfort Inn in providing a room for families in need, for the healing power of shared laughter, for the calls of support from all of our friends, for Mabel's return to care for Mom and for the blessing of a restful night's sleep. Love, Sue

DECEMBER 23, 2001

Yesterday was another peaceful day for Mom. Her vital signs remained stable through the day. She doesn't say anything, but communicates with her eyes and hand squeezes. Becky and Tom came in the morning, and stayed a while. It was fun to all sit together and remember old times. After they left, Uncle William and Aunt MM stopped by for a while. Mom knew that they were there and smiled. Laurie, a neighbor, stopped by and was able to tell Mom that she loved her and would miss her. Laurie is another example of how we are blessed with wonderful neighbors.

Diane decided that she had to get out and finish her Christmas shopping for Jenny. I sat with Mom and talked about some of the favorite recipes that Mom would prepare for us. She would acknowledge my comments, by blinking her eyes. Bryant and Jacob were also here spending time with Mom. It was hard to say good bye to Mom's nurse, Michele. Saturday was to be her last day taking care of Mom. She has been such a gift from God. I could not have done a better job taking care of Mom. She had put in some very long hours here and, not only helped with Mom, but at one point helped Diane get Ringo out of the dryer.

We were pleased, when we saw Mabel arrive at 7 p.m. We knew that we could sleep easy knowing that she was at Mom's side. All of Mom's children have been able to accept and tell Mom that we want her to have that rest that God promises all of us. I believe that Mom is still here because her heart is so strong. We don't think that she is trying to hang on out of concern for our well-being. She has not only told us, but has behaved in a way that demonstrates her desire to join her family in heaven. I said my prayers with Mom, as has been our routine. Everybody was able to sleep last night. Mabel told me that Mom also had a very restful night. The new day-nurse seems nice and our first impressions of her are good. We will have to wait and see how the day progresses.

Thank you God, for this day so sweet, for sharing memories with Tom and Becky, for Bryant and Jacob's visit with Mom, for the gift of Michele and Mabel as our Mom's nurse, for Laurie's loving words to our mother and me, for the continued calls and emails of support from all our friends and family, for Mom's smiles as we told funny stories and for one more night of a restful night's sleep. Love, Sue

DECEMBER 24, 2001

Today's note is going to be a short one. Mom had another peaceful day yesterday. She is not speaking, but interacts with us with her eyes and hand squeezes. Mom had all of her children around her bed, as the chaplain said a prayer. She had a smile on her face. I know that it was so comforting to her to have us all at her bedside at the same time. We had a caring nurse come stay with Mom for the 7 a.m. to 7 p.m. shift and also the 7 p.m. to the 7 a.m. shift. Diane and I were really able to sleep soundly.

Thank you God, for this day so sweet, for Mom's peaceful day, for the continued good nursing care, for the opportunity we had to all gather at Mom's bedside, for one more night of rest and for your peace that has replaced the fear and anxiety that had been in our hearts. Love, Sue

DECEMBER 25, 2001

Mom had a peaceful day yesterday. Her vital signs are still stable, but her breathing is more labored. We had a nurse till 10 a.m. We won't have a nurse until 7 p.m. We all are taking turns being with Mom. I am going to keep this note short today.

Thank you God, for this day so sweet, for a peaceful Christmas Eve and for the chance for all of us to gather around our mother for this last Christmas. Love, Sue

DECEMBER 26, 2001

Mom had a very peaceful Christmas. She knew that we had all gathered around her. We also told her that it was ok to let go. Her Mom and Dad were waiting to welcome her home. Mom had shopped early so she had all of our Christmas presents under the tree. I was overwhelmed with a mixture of confusing feelings. I had to laugh at one of the presents that Mom gave me. I am the proud owner of a pair of special optical glasses that allow me to lay flat in bed and be able to watch TV, with the use of special little mirrors. I think Mom heard us all thank her for all the wonderful and thoughtful gifts that she had picked out.

Mom's nurse left at 10:30, which left Diane and me to take care of Mom. Mom was in good hands, between a nurse and an accountant. Our Christmas dinner was wonderful. Jenny played a very big role in helping to pull it together. Bryant, Jacob and Sara came by early and spent time with Mom. After we had finished our lunch, Becky, Tom, Sherri and Debi came for their Christmas visit. Mom did raise her eyebrows when Diane announced, that Debi was not wearing a particular type of undergarment. We all had a laugh over her surprised response. Diane asked Tom to help figure out the problem with our deluxe electronic cat box. Something seems to always break down at Christmas.

Uncle William and Aunt MM had stopped by early in the morning on their way to Denton and came by on their way back from Denton. Uncle Dade is still hanging on and Stephen and Susanne are feeling hopeful for a recovery. They sent Mom a beautiful gardenia and a beautiful metal pole with a bird and leaves and berries wrapped around the pole. The pole is designed to hang a flower basket or a bird feeder.

Mom's night nurse returned at 7 p.m. We feel very comfortable with her. I am still so amazed that Mom is still here. Her breathing is very labored at times and her coloring will become real dusky. I did not think Mom was very responsive, but when I leaned down and told her that I loved her, she told me that she loved me. That "I love you" was the best Christmas present I could have hoped for.

After I said my prayers with Mom, I kissed her and went to bed. She had a restful night. I was so excited when I saw that Michele was back as Mom's morning nurse.

Thank you God, for this day so sweet, for the opportunity of all of us coming together to celebrate Christmas, for Jenny's corn pudding, for Mom's "I love you", for another peaceful night's sleep and for Michele's return as Mom's nurse. Love, Sue

DECEMBER 27, 2001

Mom is still with us—just barely though. Her strong heart and God's plan is the only thing that keeps her here. We have all let go and said our final good byes. For whatever reason, God has not seen fit to call her home yet. This is the hardest part of waiting and watching. She pushes the ice out of her mouth when we try to put the shaved ice in her mouth. The nurses are using little swabs to keep her mouth and tongue moist. The on-call nurse came and conferred with Michele about Mom's status and her medication. Mom's body is very stiff and she is jerking some in her sleep. After talking with the doctor, it was decided to change Mom's Roxanol (liquid morphine) to prn (as needed) because one of the side effects is muscle stiffness and jerking. They will be giving Mom a longer acting morphine in a suppository form. They also increased her topical Ativan, to help with the jerks.

Mom is still aware when we are in the room. Her eyes don't focus, but she can hear us. The phone calls and emails from family and friends are bright spots in our day. It is comforting to know that we are all surrounded with love from family and friends. I became anxious when I found out that another new nurse was coming for the 7 p.m. to 7 a.m. shift. Basically, you are expected to put a tremendous amount of faith in a stranger that an agency sends in. At night it seems so much more important to have a familiar nurse to care for Mom. Doris arrived at 7 p.m. and my first impressions of her were good. She was quiet and respectful of Mom. Michele oriented her to Mom's routine. Michele's tender and extremely competent care of our Mom, and also Mom's children, have been so deeply appreciated. It makes me proud to be a nurse. God knew that we needed Michele's gift for nursing. Before she left, Michele hugged me and told me that she thought Doris was going to be fine.

Lisa and Dria came over and brought a wonderful strawberry cake. Dria did not seem to be intimidated by Mom or our tears. She showed us how she dances like a ballerina. Their visit was enjoyed and a welcomed diversion. I went in and sat with Doris to kind of feel her out. Doris has been a nurse for 28 years and has experience in all areas of nursing, including hospice. I was telling her how worried I was that Mom would hurt unnecessarily or her mouth or tongue would dry out and cause her discomfort. I became tearful as I was talking about my fears. Doris got up and came and put her hand on my shoulder and told me that she knew how hard it was to trust a new nurse. She went on to tell me how she had cared for her mom, like I had been caring for my mom. She also struggled with having new nurses come in to care for her mom. I absolutely believed her when she assured me that she would keep Mom pain free, her mouth moist and would come and get me if there were any changes in Mom.

I went and told Diane that I felt like we had a genuine trustworthy nurse. I do have pretty good instincts about things like this. I was able to kiss Mom good night after I had said our prayers. Diane was up till around midnight. Michele was back this morning. While she was turning Mom, I put a roast on to cook, boned the turkey and put the ham bone in the freezer for a future pot of beans. I took the Christmas quilt off of Mom's bed and put on the quilt that she had made when she was ten years old.

Thank you God, for this day so sweet, for the blessings of good nursing care, for the continued support of family and friends, for morphine which eases Mom's pain, for Doris' words of comfort and for the peace that fills our hearts. Love, Sue

DECEMBER 28, 2001

Yesterday was another long day. Diane and I are in a constant state of amazement that Mom is still with us. Perhaps because she was so healthy, other than her cancer, it has been a factor in how long she has held on. I know that God will take her when it is time, but this part is so hard to watch. Her blood pressure is running around 74/54. Her eyes no longer focus. She is no longer responding to our voices. Diane and I still spend a lot of time talking with her, because hearing is the last thing to go. We are still playing her favorite hymns continuously. She is also running what they call a terminal temperature. Her thermostat is not working right. She has the sweetest set of flannel sheets on her bed. The sheets are called, "It's Raining Cats and Dogs." There are all these kittens and puppies with umbrellas. We also have the quilt she made when she was ten, on her bed. She is surrounded with all things soft, sweet and made with love.

Diane and I were sitting around Mom's bed telling "remember when" stories. Diane reminded me of the summer when I discovered that birds were having sex all over our backyard. I would come home after working 11 to 7 and look out the window and see these little sparrows fluffing out their petticoats, big black birds tumbling all over the yard (I thought they were fighting until Mom explained what was really going on.). The mourning doves were strutting, striking poses and fluffing out their feathers. I would turn to Mom and ask her to explain to me how all this worked. I had never thought of birds as having an active, healthy sex life. It was my birthday and Mom, being the consummate teacher, gave me the perfect present. She gave me a book called *How Birds Do It*.

This was a legitimate book explaining the mating habits of the bird population. I was so proud of my book. Everybody cracked up at work when I shared my bird sex book. Only my mom could find a wonderful book to explain to her adult daughter how the real birds and bees do it.

Diane and I also talked about how Mom and I combed through nurseries looking for unusual perennials to add to our garden. I told Diane that we had some flowers out there that were called Monkey Britches, Red-Hot Pokers, Turk's Cap, Bear's Britches, Lamb's Ear, Candle Tree, Purple Hyacinth Bean Vine, Cockscomb and Gay Feathers, to mention just a few of the many types of flowers that bloomed in Mom's garden. We are surrounded with so many sweet and comforting memories of how our Mother taught us about all the complexities of life. In her dying, she is still teaching. I now have no doubt that with love, and a deep personal faith, you can face seemingly insurmountable obstacles. Because my Mother shared with us how her faith and prayer saw her through each day of her life, we are able to stay and not run away from the pain of watching our mother die. Mom taught by example, and what an incredible example she was to all of us.

Bryant, Jacob and Sara came and stayed a while with Mom. Becky called frequently through the day to check on Mom. We had a wonderful surprise when Marilyn and Carol stopped by for a visit. Uncle William and Aunt MM also came by for a while. Aunt FiFi called to check on Mom. She was very tearful when she spoke of how much she will miss her sister. Uncle Dade is still in ICU and continues to be very frail. There were other supportive phone calls and emails. Doris, Mom's night nurse, came at 7 p.m. We are comforted with how she cares for our mother.

I said my prayers with Mom and turned in early for the night. Diane was up until 2 a.m. I was up at 4 a.m. The house was quiet. Mom was restless. They tell us that the jerking we see is a side effect from the high doses of morphine. I sat with Mom and told her that it was ok to let go, that she had done a good job teaching us how to take care of ourselves.

Thank you God, for this day so sweet, for all the wonders and beauty of nature, for my birds and the bees book, for another chance to sit at Mom's bedside and exchange happy memories, for Marilyn and Carol's visit, for the continued excellent nursing care and for the blessing of prayer. Love, Sue

DECEMBER 29, 2001

Yesterday was another long day. Mom is showing all the signs of terminal restlessness. She is jerking, picking at her clothes and moaning at times. The medicine does not, at this point, seem to be helping. It gets harder to watch as each hour passes. Marilyn and Carol stopped by for a brief visit. It always feels nice when they come over. Uncle William and Aunt MM also came by. Uncle William turned 84 on Friday.

Sean Mathews came over to discuss the music for Mom's funeral. He is a well-known singer in the Dallas area, and we are fortunate that he will be able to sing at Mom's funeral. Janet came by and we all gathered in Mom's room and said a prayer. I went to bed early. Diane and Jenny were awake until around 2 a.m. All of this is beginning to really wear on all of us. Prayer is certainly carrying us through. Without prayer, we would be lost trying to understand why it has to be this way for our Mother.

Thank you God, for this day so sweet, for visits from good friends, for Sean Mitchell's gift of song and for the power of prayer. Love, Sue

DECEMBER 30, 2001

Mother had a peaceful day yesterday. They have got the medicine adjusted, so she is not restless or moaning. Mom is not responsive to us. We still talk to her, in case she can still hear us. We also are still playing her hymns for her. Friends and family continue to call or come by. Becky and Tom were here and got involved in some big projects. One was putting my box spring and mattress on the floor. I wanted Grace to be able to get in bed with me and the only way it was going to happen was by putting the mattress on the floor. Becky cleaned out part of the hall closet to make room for the boxes that were under my bed. Tom and Diane worked on repairing a switch on my computer. Billy and Bryant got involved in a repair job on my toilet. It seems like it is always something. We all take turns sitting at Mom's bedside. I was restless, so I showed Jenny how to bake egg custard. Diane loves it and I thought it would be a surprise.

I said my prayers with Mom and kissed her good night. I was sure that I would be awakened and told that Mom had died. I have told myself that if I am supposed to be with Mom when she dies, then it will happen. I have to let go and trust that God will put me where I need to be. Diane stayed up until 2 a.m. I was up at 4 a.m. It is like we are sleeping in shifts.

I got the coffee made and breakfast started. The house was quiet and I was enjoying the stillness. The smell of the coffee, the hymns playing in the background and the early morning hour reminded me of mornings as a child when I would wake up and smell the coffee, hear the radio playing the hymns and Mom and Dad talking quietly. It was the safest feeling in the world. I hoped that Mom was feeling as safe and secure as I was at that moment.

Thank you God, for this day so sweet, for everybody pitching in and helping out, for Grace sleeping against my back and for sweet childhood memories. Love, Sue

DECEMBER 31, 2001

Mom died at 2:30 a.m. I had awakened at midnight and was restless, so I spent time with Mom. I had just stepped out of the room at 2:30, when the nurse called me and I looked and saw that Mom had stopped breathing. Diane, Jenny and I bathed Mom and dressed her in a pretty nightgown and socks with flowers. Bryant was also here to say his good byes. I called Becky earlier to let her know.

Sparkman Hillcrest is doing the funeral. There will be visitation on Wednesday at 7 p.m. at Sparkman. The funeral will be at Westminister Presbyterian Church on Devonshire at 10 a.m. on Thursday. We will then go to Cleburne for the grave side service and burial. If you can come, please do. We would love to see all of you.

Thank you God, for this day so sweet and for blessing us with such a remarkable mother. Love, Sue

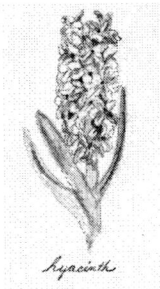

hyacinth

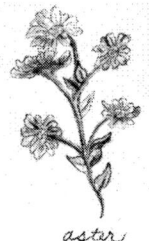

aster

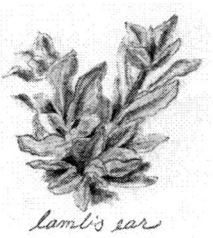

lamb's ear

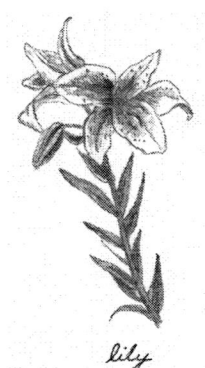

lily

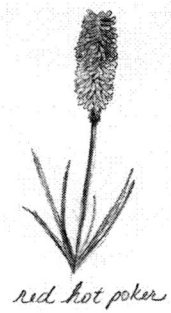

red hot poker

PART TWO
SUE

AFTER THE FUNERAL, Sue continued to live in her mother's house. The day before Sally's funeral Grace Elizabeth had a grand mal seizure. She passed away three months later. Sue continued on, with the cats as her companions. Due to the progression of her idiopathic pulmonary fibrosis she was confined to her bedroom most of the time and unable to walk due to her breathlessness. She was house-bound the entire next year, except for one trip to the bank to give Diane access to Sue's accounts.

She did come out of her room for Christmas that year, 2002. Diane and Jenny drove up to spend it with her. Diane had a shattered ankle and Jenny was unable to maintain balance because of a brain tumor. Sue looked at them all, as she stood at the sink preparing Christmas dinner, and said, "My God, I am the healthiest person in this house- and I'm dying."

What follows are the last messages from Sue from the time she was admitted to hospice care.

OCT 16, 2002

I had a somewhat restless night. I would guess that officially becoming a patient of hospice has been assuming different sizes and shapes, with some of them comforting, and then some leaving me with a frightened feeling. Ringo decided to be very snuggly with me and commenced to wrap his 2x sized body around my head like a turban. Those of you that have had the opportunity to gaze upon the large and lovely cat can really appreciate his contortions at 5 a.m. I quickly completed my morning kitty routine and returned to burrow down in my bed.

Not long after my morning routine of checking fluid levels and making adjustments to the type and amount of fuel that my body requires for the day, I have spoken to Becky and Cil, and my day has officially begun. Bryant and Monica soon arrive. He wants to be here when hospice arrives to do their admission assessment. Lynda stopped by to have lunch. She had made meatloaf sandwiches. Lunch doesn't get much better than this. We chatted and giggled about things at work.

As Lynda was leaving, Mike stopped by to look at the new walking sticks that Bryant has carved. Soon after he arrived I experienced the biggest treat and surprise. Cil and Delbert were at my front door, with a big catfish grins on their faces. After all the hugs, kisses and squeals of delight, we all had to sit down and catch our breath. Paratta, my friend, had sent me a wondrous green frog that was made for snuggling. Cil had picked out a plush Santa and Mrs. Santa that played music. She knows how I love Santas. She had also included Avon's Superlube for lips in need. My lips are certainly in need from the wind shear that my fan produces.

Before too long it was time to say goodbye to Delbert and Cil. Bryant and Monica had already left for home. I climbed into bed with my lips super-lubed and a frog to hold against my chest. It did not appear that, for whatever reason, hospice will come today. I was tired, so it was just as well that they did not come today. I was treated to a phone call from Lynda while she was on her break. While I was going through my nightly routine, Becky called to make sure all was well. I had an absolutely delightful day filled with friends, family laughter and gifts that had love written all over them.

After such a full day, it did not take long to get through my bedtime routine and have myself tucked in tight for the night.

Thank you God for this day so sweet, for a cat's different way of communicating their needs, for sharing giggles and a homemade meatloaf sandwich with Lynda, for Cil and Delbert and Paratta and how much richer, interesting and joyful life has become since they became a part of my life. Love, Sue

OCT 24, 2002

Pat is a good friend and neighbor

Hello All,

It has been a while since I have written. I had hoped to be able to write every day. It seems as though I will have to go with the flow. I am really battling the fatigue and shortness of breath whenever I move.

Kathy came Thursday to finish up the nursing assessment. It was so good to see her. She was Mom's nurse and I have kept in touch with her through email. Instead of VS vicodin that I have been taking for headaches and back pain, she asked me to try liquid morphine. She also said they have a way for me to use a nebulizer set up, that will allow me to inhale morphine into my lungs. This is supposed to be very helpful with the shortness of breath.

Thursday was a pretty quiet day for me. I am sleeping pretty well at night. Lynda came over and surprised me with the thin magical pillow case for my old neck pillow that has become like a security blanket. She ran some errands for me and picked up some videos and groceries. We had a good time talking and laughing.

My morning and evening phone routines are still a part of every day. Marion, the social worker, called and wanted to see me Friday afternoon. We had to plan to get together on Monday because I had an appointment with the doctor on Friday. I had to call and cancel the appointment with the doctor because of how I felt and the weather was terrible. Before I know it, Saturday has arrived and Becky is coming to my house to work her special kind of magic. She has picked up some groceries for me and surprised me with several new frozen soups and with a wonderful carrot raisin salad. She also had made some of Mom's fruitcake cookies for me and had baked a coconut pound cake for Lynda.

After she had freshened the house, it was time for my hair cut. I always get sleepy when I am in the process of getting a hair cut and Becky starts chatting. I find myself smiling as I start to get sleepy and hear Becky chatting. I have many memories of some of her marathon talking. Becky was soon headed back to Bedford and I was tucked in for the night.

Ringo woke me at 5 a.m. and insisted that I get up and feed him. He would rake his paw down the wooden blinds and then turn around to see if I was moving. I finally gave in to his demands.

I am not sure why, but Sunday was a difficult day for me to get a deep breath. Early Sunday morning I took my first dose of liquid morphine. Initially I was not really feeling the effects of the morphine. I can have it every two hours. I took a second dose two hours later and began to feel some easing of my shortness of breath. Sunday was a long day for me. It seemed that it was a struggle to accomplish anything, other than trying to lay still with my head centered in front of the fan.

Frankly, I wondered if I had really started sliding. The doctor told me on September 17th that I had six months or so left to live. That was about two months and two weeks ago. There is so much left that I not only need to do, but I want to do. I need to see Tom one more time.

Sunday afternoon Pat came over and did a little of picking up and corralling the kitties, in addition to cleaning their deluxe cat box. We watched a Bloopers Show she had taped earlier. I felt so blessed as she helped me with my medicine, and preparing my dinner along with getting my water bottles and diet Big Red set up by my bed. As I said good night to Pat the phone was ringing and Cil was calling to wish me sweet dreams. We had talked several times during the day about how powerless one can feel when they are trying to control the panic you feel when you are having to struggle for the next breath. Becky also called to say goodnight. She knew it was almost time for the *Sopranos*. I was all tucked in for the night, but my focus was in New Jersey with the Soprano family.

The next thing I knew, it was 5:15 and Ringo was strumming the blinds. He persuaded me to get up in five minutes and lay out their breakfast buffet. Pat came and surprised me with some wonderful scrambled eggs and toast.

Around 11 a.m. Kathy, my nurse, called and asked me if I would enjoy hearing someone sing me a pretty song. The Director of Volunteers soon arrived with Stephanie. Stephanie had an incredible voice and loved to sing the old hymns. She sang *I'll Fly Away* and *Just a Closer Walk With Thee* and *Jesus Loves Me*. She said she would come back and sing more songs. We all spent some time chatting before they had to leave.

It is 4 p.m. on Monday and I am going to end this note with plans to begin another note tomorrow. I do wish that I could promise a note every day, but I can't. I also want to thank everyone for all the wonderful notes of support.

Thank you God, for this world so sweet, for a nurse named Kathy, for my wonderful magical flannel pillow case that has pictures of sock monkeys, cats and penguins, for Becky and the way she comes in with her special ways of putting the house right, for Glade Apple Cinnamon Scented plug ins, sweet childhood memories, for the relief that liquid morphine brings me, for all the phone calls, for the Sopranos, for Pat making me a wonderful breakfast of scrambled eggs and toast, for Stephanie sharing her gift of song with me. Love, Sue

OCT 24, 2002

When I fell asleep Wednesday night, I had no idea of what was in store for me. I have two large one hundred gallon tanks that hold my liquid oxygen. They are rather large and intimidating. When I first saw these tanks, I thought of cryogenics and how Walt Disney decided to be preserved through cryogenics. Becky wandered in the room and I told her I think that the tank on the right was where old Walt Disney was hanging. She shook her head "no" and declared that I was crazy. I told her that she could not prove he wasn't in there, and besides, I thought it was kind of neat thinking about having a little bit of Disney in my home.

Anyhow, I woke at 2:30 a.m. and could not breathe. I checked both tanks and they were both empty. I immediately began to focus on controlling my rising panic. I was able to call Cil and Delbert for help. Delbert arrived within thirty minutes with two portable tanks of oxygen. Seeing Delbert carrying those tanks toward me was much like watching a fireman carrying a child out of a burning building. I dozed off for a while, then I woke and put in an emergency call to Dallas Life Support. I also called Pat and asked her if she could come and feed Max and Ringo. I was way past being exhausted. Soon I had a third tank added to my oxygen supply and sweet Pat had fed the cats and me.

Well, let me get back to Wednesday. I spoke to all my family and friends in addition to reading all my wonderful emails. I have enjoyed the notes that have updates about what was happening in their families. My cousin, Lily, has written me several times about the comings and goings in her family. I also enjoy the jokes, cartoons and assorted stories. Monica and her friend, Matt, stopped by for a visit. It felt good that Monica independently wanted to come and visit me. The hospice admission nurse, Pat, called to say that she would be here around noon to begin the admission process for hospice. Lynda is also coming over for lunch and we are having chili dogs with Fritos. Pat commented on how rare it was to have had a mother in their care a year earlier and to be admitting her daughter the next year. I decided to choose the same hospice because of how close we had grown to her caregivers. I am sure I will feel like I have family watching over me.

Lynda and I polished off the chili dogs while I was answering Pat's questions. Pat had said "no thanks" to the chili dogs. We finished up and it was time for Pat to go to her next patient, and Lynda needed to go to work. I decided it was time to snuggle down in bed for a while.

The salesman from Hoveround scooters called and told me that he would be delivering my Hoveround Thursday. I napped on and off the rest of the afternoon. I would get up and type one or two lines and then would go lay down. I was feeling real sleepy. I decided to dine on grilled chicken breasts along with a baked potato. I swear, I don't think I ever got out of first gear today. I told Becky, Bryant, Cil and Diane good night. I had finished lubricating all exposed skin to prevent any frostbite during the night.

Thank you God, for this day so sweet, for the visit with Monica and Matt, for the wonder of email, for the chance to eat chili dogs and Fritos with my friend Lynda, for baked potatoes, for the feeling of anticipation of what another day will bring, for Cil and Delbert being there for me at 2:30 in the morning and for being able to take a deep satisfying breath, courtesy of Delbert, my hero. Love, Sue

OCT 24, 2002

My last note covered my time up to 4 p.m. on Monday. Marion, the hospice social worker, came by for a visit Monday afternoon. We talked about Do Not Resuscitate, Durable Power of Attorney, my will, my ability to care for myself now and in the future, and when I would be weaker and in need of someone available all the time. I was not overwhelmed with sadness, but felt an urgency to put things in order so that I did not have my time occupied with technical legal things.

This week it felt like I was picking up some speed as I rolled down the hill. This getting weaker is for the birds. I did find the strength to play with Max while I was in bed. She loves this stick with a string attached to it. She was hopping, romping and scampering as we played. That time was very good for both of us.

Tuesday began, as it typically does, with Ringo playing "it is breakfast time" on the wooden blinds around 5:15 a.m., followed by Becky's phone call around 6, followed by a phone call from Cil around 8, and followed by a call from Pat, around 8 and 10. Pat then comes over and prepares me a wonderful breakfast. I think that it is true; toast does taste better when someone else toasts the bread. Pat's way of toasting the bread far exceeds the toasts I have had in the past. Other family and friends will often call between the other calls, not to mention all the wonderful emails and greeting cards. Lynda has been stopping by around noon, with a surprise lunch before she is on her way to work a 3 to 11 shift. I decided to ask Lynda how peculiar a question sounded to her—I had this cross my mind and it had me laughing out loud. But it sounded kind of morbid. I knew she was going to scream, but I went on and asked her, "Do they have chubby sized coffins?" I mean is it like a dress, where the sizes go from petit to plus size, or is it like Burger King, where you can have your order Super-sized? Needless to say, she started whooping and slapping her leg. I asked her what she thought would happen when I added this to observations that I send out to family and friends. She told me she was sure folks would let me know.

My nurse, Kathy, came by to check me out on using the nebulized morphine. And she just laughed and told me my sense of humor was in high gear. Taking the morphine by nebulizer was helpful, but initially caused a little coughing. I think it will be very helpful. Lisa and Joe, my neighbors, are back in town and they called to check on me. Bryant and Monica checked in on me. Monica's daily emails have also been a part of my routine.

Wednesday I had my water bottle loaded and prepared to do battle with Ringo's sense of timing. Sure enough, 5:15 a.m. rolled around and he began doing his morning thang. I shot him a few times and then he moved to a blind behind me where I nailed him with water. Then he finally moved to under my desk and started kicking up there. Well, I finally ran him out of the room with my ability to shoot regular, underhand, behind me and over my shoulder. I did eventually get up and feed him, but Ringo didn't even say good morning before he began banging out his tune. Max is always polite and never forgets his manners, when it comes to meal time.

Pat came this morning to tend to the kitties and me. Lynda surprised me again with lunch. I felt a little out of focus today, because I had to use a little more morphine to deal with my shortness of breath. Lynda stopped by with another surprise lunch of barbecue, cole slaw and baked beans. It had been so long since I had eaten barbecue that I had forgotten how much I enjoy the flavors. She then topped it off with an early Christmas present. My eyes were closed when she handed me the gift. It was my time to hoop and holler. Lynda had given me a hardback book all about the Sopranos and the Mob. I had a grin on my face that resisted any attempts to achieve a normal, less crazed look. After Lynda had left for work, my face began to calm down. I met Brenda, my personal care assistant from hospice. She seems nice and her help will be welcomed. I dozed off and on the rest of the afternoon. Lisa called and asked me if I would enjoy some grilled chicken. Lisa is a wonderful cook and is the mother of two beautiful little girls. I was not long for bed after eating dinner.

Thursday morning's attempt by Ringo to express himself was extinguished fairly quickly. It looked like I was going to have a fairly quite day. I was expecting to have my oxygen tanks filled up. I was pleasantly surprised when Marilyn called and wanted to stop by for a visit. She came bearing wonderful containers filled with homemade food. I could not tell you exactly what we talked about, but I was left wrapped securely with such warmth and comfort. Lynda whipped by on her way to work to pick up some movies to return. Everybody called to check in on me. I was really ready for my bedtime routine and prayers.

Thank you God, for this day so sweet, for people that are good at organizing papers and taking pity on and helping those people who haven't a clue, for Ringo and his personality, even the part that wakes me at 5 a.m., for an intense thirty minute filled time playing with Max and his stick with some string on it, for having friends that enjoy cooking and who know where the good stuff can be found, for the gifts of seeing Dria wearing her yellow Snow White shoes with the red bows, and Adeline showing me how she is beginning to crawl, for the email about the man super glued to his recliner for three days and the laughter that is still felt when I think about it, for the peace that comes with prayer, for the chance to see Sue walk Rusty, he is a wondrous dog that makes you want to smile real big, for moms like Lisa that understand the importance of shoes matching your attitude. Love, Sue

OCTOBER 25, 2002
*Sue is trying to be admitted to a clinical trial of actimmune,
a new medicine which could possibly help her condition*

Good Morning, Good Morning,

I woke early this morning and thought I would touch base with all of you. Yesterday was a long day of waiting to hear from Parkland. I did call in the afternoon and there is still no decision as to an appointment, much less the medication. I will call again today.

I was surprised when Lynda stopped by around 11 a.m. with some tuna from Subway. I was surprised primarily because I am sleeping during the day. In the past, when I woke up for the day, I was awake. I guess something has shifted inside and I am doing some power napping.

Cil and Delbert stopped by and brought one of her wheelchairs for me to use when I get out. Having the use of her chair will allow me to go on and get the Hoverround. It will be helpful in the house. I am beginning to get short of breath when I walk a few feet, so the little scooter chair will take me any place I want to go. I did spend some time on the Actimmune site and found the list of all the folks that run the company, from the CEO to the pharmacist. I am thinking about composing a letter to the CEO about my precarious position. In addition, I thought that I could send copies of the letter to the *Dallas Morning News*, TV stations, government officials and anybody else any of you can think of.

Pat stopped by after work and tended to my kitties. She has been a faithful friend and neighbor. I will be getting blood work done today. I hope it is a little dryer outside.

Thank you God, for this day so sweet, phone calls and emails from my sisters, brother and nieces, surprise visits from Lynda and the wonderful subway sandwiches, watching John Fogerty on DVD, Christmas catalogues in the mail, finding the plastic bugs, snakes and scorpions, that Becky so lovingly planted around my room, the cool weather, my wonderful fan (although I am probably going to have to contact Chapstick and see if they make a big whole body Chapstick. I am having to keep my eyes and nose lubricated. There are many challenges one faces, when they live in a wind tunnel), wonderful steak dinner, courtesy of Tom and Becky, the sweet comfort of home. Love, Sue

OCTOBER 26, 2002

Good Morning,

My morning started as it has for some time now. I get an early phone call from Becky. The cats have been sitting in the green chair staring at me. They are waiting for me to feed them. This is usually followed by a call from Cil. We compare our breathing with what is going on with the weather. I am also able to do this with Bryant. My good friend and neighbor, Pat, calls to check in and see if the kitties or I need anything. Often she will come in the morning and take care of the cat box and any other chore that would be helpful to me. She sometimes comes again in the evening. From my bed, I can see the comings and goings of Joe, Lisa and the kids. From my front window I can catch Sue walking Rusty. I spend time checking blood sugars and calculate my insulin dosage for the morning. Breakfast was simple and I went on and took the rest of my morning meds. After all of this, I am back in bed with the covers pulled up.

Lynda, Becky and Bryant all called wanting to know if Parkland had called. Well, I called Parkland again and was told to check back on Monday. The head of the department had not yet reached a decision. I refuse to give in and give them my interpretation of Chicken Little on steroids. All I would accomplish is scaring them and having a referral to the psychiatric department. I did speak to two pulmonologists in Austin and Houston about ongoing clinical trials with Actimmune. I was told that it was a two year study and they did not have any vacancies. I did get a chance to speak to Diane and she volunteered to write the letter to the president of Actimmune with copies going to newspapers, TV stations, government officials and whoever else we can think of. The biggest obstacle I am confronted with is the extreme fatigue. I needed to go to Dr. H's office to have blood work done and I could not get myself pulled together. After turning my oxygen up to 6 ¾ liters, I was able to shower and change clothes. After my shower, I called Dr. H's office and asked that they have a home health nurse come on Monday to draw my blood.

I was surprised by a visit from Sue. She came bearing a gift and a funny, funny card. I am now styling with a new toe ring and ankle bracelet. We sat and talked and shared some really wonderful, deep laughs. The kind of laughs, that make you feel so alive and connected to the world.

Dr. M called as I was saying good bye to Sue. We talked for a while about the degree of fatigue I was feeling. I told him that I did not think it was depression. He told me that if someone had told him that he was dying that he would be shitting in his pants. I paused for a moment, and told him that I was really, really hoping that in this journey I am on, I would not have to experience the "pant's shitting" part of it. We both laughed at where the conversation had taken us. In talking with him, I was aware of how my feelings about dying changes from feeling like I am watching this happen to someone else, and then, at times, I am acutely aware of the feeling of life slipping away. Like I said, when I wrote about Mom, I am going to write about even the scary parts. It makes it less scary to put my thoughts and experiences in the light and also to share them with those that I love.

Becky's plastic snake that she gave to me in the hospital—I know, I know, instead of flowers, she brings rubber snakes, pointy toed, eye gouging Poinsettia fairies, and my mother's robe for me to snuggle with because she thought the smell from Mom's robe would comfort me. How sweet is that? It still brings a tear to my eye. What is not to love about having a sister that thinks like Becky does? Excuse the rambling, I wanted to describe an incident in my room with this pesky rubber snake. Someone had placed the snake on top of my large, liquid oxygen tank. It happened to be laying on this tip where the oxygen comes out. I looked over at the tank and saw a snowball with a snake in the middle of the snowball. I almost did not believe my eyes. I had to scrape away the ice to keep the oxygen from leaking out.

I have spent a major portion of my day in bed. I am hoping that Saturday will be the day I am able to make it out of the house. I have not been out of the house since I came home from the hospital. I guess I am getting cabin fever. I enjoyed one of Tom's wonderful steaks for dinner. Pat stopped by with a Friday paper for me and we visited for a while and we also shared a laugh. She locked up the house for the night and I made my evening phone calls. I checked in with Becky, Bryant and Cil and we all exchange wishes for sweet dreams.

Thank you God, for this day so sweet, for morning phone calls from people that I love, really good soft scrambled eggs, with pepper jack cheese, for Diane and her desire to fight for me with her talent for letter writing, shared laughter, Tom's steak dinner, the chance to wish those I love "Sweet Dreams" and a sister named Becky, that brings me the gift of a rubber snake. Love, Sue

OCTOBER 27, 2002
Good Morning to all,

Saturday started slowly for me. I know for a fact that it really irritates Ringo that there is so much time between when I open my eyes, to sitting upright, and finally, having food in his bowl and the backdoor opened so he can have his time to stalk any frog, lizard or unattractive bug that happens to be walking in his kingdom. Max is always happy when I fill her food bowl. After she eats, she is more interested in having her tummy tickled. I identify with how Max feels about people tickling her tummy. I have a spot on my right shoulder that is always begging to be scratched. Mother scratching my back is something I truly miss. I am not above having friends or strangers, yes strangers, scratch my right shoulder. Like Max, I figure if they aren't driving, eating or writing, they have a free hand that could be used for a very good purpose. Max does not require any introductions. She will tiptoe in and stretch out on her back waiting for her tummy to be tickled. She points her toes, like I do when folks tickle or scratch in just the right way. Max sadly points out that if she had not been declawed, that she could give me a good back scratch. This causes me to think how important it is that we really think before we permanently alter our bodies.

I wasn't planning on getting on my soapbox, but I don't resist where my mind takes me. This is for all my nieces and maybe one sister. No more piercing or tattoos. I speak from life experiences about one's body being like the Sahara desert. It is continually changing shape. The sand, like your body, will suddenly flatten out on you, mounds or strange formations are formed like speed bumps, and the mounds are never where it would be a benefit. There can even be the dreaded cave in, or an oasis dries up and becomes a mirage, not to mention the splotches of brown on your skin, courtesy of hormones and the sun. A tattoo of a little heart on your shoulder could end up on a hump on your neck, and then people are whispering about why anybody would tattoo the buffalo hump on their neck. I know, I can hear each of you say that you would never have a hump on your neck, much less one that the medical community refers to as a "buffalo hump." Mamaw feet, I don't think I will go into the horror of Mamaw feet today, but I will later. Just know that I went to work one night and everything was just fine. By the next morning, I was on the phone talking with my sister and looked down and started screaming into the phone "Mamaw feet!...Mamaw feet!"

I think it would only be fair if our bodies gave us a warning, like geologists do when they feel like California is on the verge of becoming an island, or some volcano that had been quiet for centuries was going to begin to spew hot lava and rock. It would be wonderful to be given, say 5 days, then this body part was going to disappear and reappear in a place that makes all your clothes fit funny. All to say, treasure your body and think of it like a map, with new continents being discovered, communities and neighborhoods evolving. There might be a San Andreas Fault in your future.

Anyhow back to my day, I was able to pull myself together. Pat joined me for my first outing. We made it to the Video Store and I was only able to walk a short distance before I had to call it quits. I was a little surprised that I was so weak and that I wasn't able to make my body respond to my demands. It is a sense of a very real and most intimate betrayal when you no longer are able to make your body respond to your demands. Being humbled is a word that comes to mind in thinking of my body beginning to fail me. We did go to Tom Thumb and Pat brought one of the motorized scooters to the car for me. I can't remember the last time that I had been to the store. I had a wonderful time cruising up and down the aisles. Pat was so wonderful and patient with me.

After our outing, I came in and poured myself into bed! Pat brought in all the groceries, put them up, fed the cats and baked a potato for me. Pat certainly exemplifies what it means to be a good friend and a good neighbor. I let Cil and Becky know that I was home and tucked into bed. I was pleasantly surprised when Monica and Bryant came by for a visit. We chatted a while in the kitchen, then I told them that I was going to have to go lay down. As I snuggled down in bed I could hear them talking to each other. I can't begin to describe how warm and comforting it was to listen to them as I drifted off to sleep. I had a good night's sleep.

Thank you God, for this day so sweet, for the mysteries of cats, finding someone with a hand available for tickling or scratching, for store scooters, for a friend and neighbor named Pat, for the sweet comfort of familiar family voices and for taking away my Mamaw feet and giving me back girl feet. Love, Sue

OCTOBER 27, 2002
Good Morning All,

I had a night full of dreams. While I was waking, I would have sworn that I could smell my Mother's comfort-cooking smells and felt Gracie at my back always watching and taking care. As I became fully awake, I was left with wonderful memories and feelings. I am not sure why there are other times that those same memories would bring a tear to my eye. I would imagine that is the nature of grief and the healing process.

The kitties were more patient with me this morning. It felt so wonderful, when I opened the back door for Ringo and felt how cool it was outside. Ringo turned to Max and asked her if I was getting ready to scamper. Max assured Ringo that there would be some heartfelt scampering the first time there was a frost. I can hardly wait for that time. I finished up in the kitchen and headed back to the comfort of my room and bed. I quickly moved through the glucose testing, and the taking of the pills. Becky's morning call was welcome. After chatting with Becky, I called Cil to see how her night was.

I am deeply thankful for the routine exchange of phone calls with family and friends. Routines, at times, I think are underestimated. A seemingly brief morning phone call encompasses me with the certainty and security of being loved, which carries over to the exchange of phone calls in the evening full of prayers for a peaceful night's rest.

I spent most of the day in bed. I found myself napping and then waking up to see if there was anything amazing on TV, like funny animal videos, shows about organized crime, ice skating, Classic Westerns and anything to do with the Civil War. Pat came over later in the day and we watched a western on my new DVD player. I showed off a little by predicting what was going to happen next. I had not seen the movie, but geeeeeze, I have put in a lot of time with the TV, so hopefully I have learned something.

I did learn an unpleasant fact about TV watching. I thought only people typing on a keyboard got carpal tunnel syndrome-NOT SO! Excessive use, or misuse, of the remote control can lead to carpal tunnel. Folks are not really sympathetic to carpal tunnel syndrome secondary to a remote control.

After Pat left for home, Lynda called and she was relieved to have all the necessary information to begin her orientation at Timberlawn on Monday. I was officially tucked into bed and was ready for the Sopranos on HBO. Sunday was a warm snugly kind of day. Becky and Tom were home safe, after going to Denton to share an early birthday celebration with Stephen and FiFi. I talked with Diane and all was well in Beaumont.

Thank you God, for this day so sweet, for dreams and warm memories, for the healing process of grief, for routines, for my carpal tunnel improving with better positioning of the remote control in my hand and for the gift of your love and the love of my family and friends. Love, Sue

OCTOBER 28, 2002
Good Morning All,

Last night was a fair night. Ringo and Max were surprised when I snuck out of bed at 4:30 a.m. to feed them. It is hard to sneak up on a cat. Anyway, I kept finding and then losing the sweet spot in bed. You will not only find sweet spots in older beds. You can also find dangerous abandoned mines, land fills, steep slopes and rough terrains in an old mattress. I have an old double sized striped mattress on my antique bed that requires careful placements of blankets under the mattress to prevent me from sliding off of the precipice, otherwise known as the edge of the mattress. I now sleep on a single hospital bed. In an attempt to make it more comfortable, I have put a special foam mattress on it that I have had for some years. I bought it six or seven years ago when I was going through my home shopping network phase. The mattress cost me about $300 and originally was a Queen Size. When Mom and I combined households and I was the proud new owner of my antique bed I was faced with a dilemma. I loved my foam mattress, but it was too big for the bed. I found myself standing in my room at the end of a long exhausting day and Becky was holding a pair of giant pair of razor sharp scissors and I was going to have to decide whether or not I was going to give my permission to cut the foam to fit my bed. After all the cutting, Grace and I made a horrible discovery. The bed was, on its own, very high off of the floor. The mattress and the foam mattress combined had me not only at a precarious nose bleed elevation, but Grace risked being catapulted off of the bed and embedded into the bedroom wall if I innocently turned in my sleep.

Time has passed and now I am presented with the twin sized electric hospital bed, the double sized foam mattress and Becky with Razor Sharp Shears. They are the kind of scissors that, at first glance, would cause any young man to pass out from the fear of such a sight, not to mention, cause a young male sheep or young bull to cry out for their mother. When you see my old foam mattress, you see mountains and valleys. In order to try and get any comfort left in that old foam mattress, you have to tie the sheets on the bed in a very tight manner. I think of it like I am putting a long line girdle on my bed. The sheets hold the mattress and foam mattress for maybe a day, then things start to shift and move. Half of the foam mattress has moved to the underside of the bed. Soon, and I do mean soon, I am getting a brand new temperpedic mattress that is all business and no hidden sweet spots. Enough about the dangers of mattresses.

I promised Becky that I would call Parkland by 11 a.m. to see if I could get an appointment time with a pulmonologist to get started on Actimmune. Pat was here running the vacuum. I finally got a response from the head nurse of the chest clinic. I was told that the head of pulmonology would not ok dispensing any Actimmune for me. She said that they had just finished a clinical trial and had no plans at this time for any further studies. I finally got my answer.

After hanging up, I felt like I had just had the wind knocked out of me. A few tears were shed. Everything in my life had shifted just a little bit. The tears did not last long. I knew that I was going to contact hospice about becoming one of their patients. I called my family and friends. Diane was scared that I was giving up. I assured her that I was not giving up, but while we were looking for funding, I could benefit from the care that hospice provided. I also let her know that I would need much more time in preparing for my departure. Like I haven't figured out how I could make contact with her at her house without all of her cats taking credit for my reaching out to touch her. Cats have a reputation of being mysterious and always get blamed for unexplainable events in a home. Diane was able to chuckle about her cats.

Hospice assured me that I could have the same chaplain, nurse and social worker. It all seems like a strange coincidence that Mother was admitted to their care at the end of August or first of September. A year later, I find myself in need of their care.

Everybody checked in and wanted to help. I was in ok shape and wished all sweet dreams. After I was tucked in for the night, I found myself watching *Birth Day* on the Discovery Channel. On one of the shows they had midwives attending the women in their homes. I am attracted to that and the show *Trading Places*. I will need to think on that for a while.

Thank you God, for this day so sweet, for sweet spots, for hospice, for the reassurances from family and friends that you are loved, for your sweet, sweet peace, that fills my soul and for that old foam mattress. Love, Sue

---

IN AUGUST OF 2003 SUE CALLED her sister Diane and asked if she could come to Diane's house to live. Diane arranged to have two special huge tanks of oxygen placed in her car so that she and Sue could make the trip. They drove to Beaumont, Texas. Sue moved into Diane's large bedroom where she lived the last twelve weeks of her life. She died on Monday, November 17th.

The day that she died, Sue woke up with a pain in her shoulder. Diane said, "Maybe you slept on it wrong," and rubbed it for her, but that didn't help. They thought it might be an upper respiratory infection. Sue was uncharacteristically quiet all day. Diane fed her a few bites but she wasn't herself. Diane called the hospice nurse and asked her to come. The nurse told Diane to give Sue morphine, but Diane said, "No, you need to come." Diane was in another room and she heard Sue's breathing change. She got up and by the time she had walked into the bedroom, Sue was gone.

Sue's niece, Sherri, once asked Sue if she were afraid of dying. Sue looked at her and said, "Honey, I can't worry about dying...that would cut into my TV time."

Beaumont, Texas 77706
November 18, 2003

Blue Bell Creameries
Consumer Relations
P.O. Box 1807
Brenham, TX 77833

Dear Blue Bell,

My sister, Sally Sue Tittle, loved your Homemade Vanilla ice cream. She was such a fan that she instructed my daughter, Jenny, to give out gift certificates for Blue Bell at her funeral, so that she could share with her friends and family.

Tonight Sue lost her battle with Pulmonary Fibrosis and passed away. I haven't been able to go to sleep; my heart is hurting. I thought that I would write to you and see if I could find out if, and how, I might get gift certificates for her funeral. Could you please advise me of the best way to do this?

Thank you,

Diane Baxter

Order Form

To order additional copies
please send $15.00 plus $4.00 shipping and handling to
A WING AND A PRAYER PRESS
PO BOX 550,
SEABECK, WA 98380
Please enclose check or money order.

Name: _____

Address: _____

City: _____ State: _____ Zip: _____

Phone: _____

e-mail: _____

Or visit our website at
www.awingandaprayerpress.com